VETERAN'S PTSD HANDBOOK

D0509261

Also by John D. Roche

The Veteran's Survival Guide

Roche, John D., Maj.
The veteran's PTSD
handbook : how to file a
c2007.
33305213022217
mi   01/23/08

THE
VETERAN'S
PTSD
HANDBOOK

How to File and Collect on Claims for Post-traumatic Stress Disorder

John D. Roche

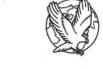

POTOMAC BOOKS, INC.
WASHINGTON, D.C.

Copyright © 2007 John D. Roche

Published in the United States by Potomac Books, Inc. All rights reserved. No part of this book may be reproduced in any manner whatsoever without written permission from the publisher, except in the case of brief quotations embodied in critical articles and reviews.

Library of Congress Cataloging-in-Publication Data
Roche, John D., Maj.
  The veteran's PTSD handbook : how to file and collect on claims for post-traumatic stress disorder / John D. Roche. — 1st ed.
    p. ; cm.
  Includes bibliographical references and index.
  ISBN-13: 978-1-59797-064-8 (alk. paper)
  1. Post-traumatic stress disorder. 2. Veterans—Legal status, laws, etc. 3. Veterans—Psychology. 4. Military pensions. I. Title.
  [DNLM: 1. Stress Disorders, Post-Traumatic—United States. 2. Veterans Disability Claims—legislation & jurisprudence—United States. 3. Veterans—psychology—United States. W 32.5 AA1 R673va 2006]

  RC552.P67R63 2006
  616.85'21008697—dc22
                                        2006018027

Printed in the United States of America on acid-free paper that meets the American National Standards Institute Z39-48 Standard.

Potomac Books, Inc.
22841 Quicksilver Drive
Dulles, Virginia 20166

First Edition

10 9 8 7 6 5 4 3 2 1

We drifted o'er the harbour-bar, And I with sobs did pray
O let me be awake, my God! Or let me sleep always."
— Samuel Taylor Coleridge, *The Rime of the Ancient Mariner*

CONTENTS

PREFACE

Several events led me to resign as a Department of Veterans Affairs (VA) adjudicator and become a veterans' advocate. After leaving the U.S. Air Force, I became a claims examiner for the VA. It wasn't long before I learned that there was a definite bureaucratic pecking order. As the new kid on the block, I had difficulty learning how not to transgress these protocols.

Mr. GS-13

Under no circumstance does one respond to criticism from a GS-13 section chief. To do so is to cause a bureaucratic firestorm. Here's what happened to elevate me to top of the "watch your step" list. Mr. GS-13 was a very proper man who wore his importance with considerable pride. Career advancement hinged on his perception of your worth. I'll let you judge how serious my indiscretion was to rocket me to the head of the list.

All was great with my world; the pay was good, my kids were all in school and had realistic goals, and our house made the front cover of *Scott's Fertilizer* magazine thanks to my wife. That was until 12:35 PM one Tuesday in August.

Having enjoyed my thirty-minute lunch break, plus a five-minute bathroom break, I was all set to do good for our veterans. As I walked to my desk, I discovered Mr. GS-13 charging down the aisle like "Storming Norman" of the first Persian Gulf War fame. As I watched the distance between us shrink, I asked myself "what did I do *now*?"

"Mr. Roche, why is it necessary for me to remind you that lunch is from 12:00 to 12:30, not till 12:35?" The entire section became quiet while waiting to see what would happen next. I answered back in equal volume, "Well, Mr. GS-13, the government allowed me to drink water on government time so I just figured it was all right to pee on government time." When the entire section started to snicker, Mr. GS-13 retreated back to his "office" (really a cubicle) in a foul mood. My section mates also received his caustic wrath that afternoon.

I further alienated myself from Mr. GS-13 when I continuously exceeded the twenty-five cases per day performance standard. There are days when cases are resolved one, two, three. This time, Mr. GS-13 wasn't going to chat with me before an audience. I was invited back to his cubicle where he advised me it was not in the VA's best interest for me to exceed the twenty-five cases-per-day work standard. He pointed out that the division received its manpower and budget authorization based on a twenty-five-case-per-day standard. If I continued to turn out more cases than the standard, I could upset the budget and manpower allocations set for this division.

"But, sir," I replied, "I really think I'm helping you because my extra cases per day will pick up the slack when some of my colleagues fail to reach their twenty-five-case-per-day quotas." He said in a tone that could only be read as "failure to obey would bring down the bureaucratic gods who will dispatch you to somewhere other than to the land of VA Oz." He actually said, "There is no debate here, Mr. Roche, do you understand?" "Yes, sir. I will do only twenty-five cases each day and I will finish the last one by 4:28 PM each workday." I really needed the two extra minutes to make my work zone shipshape before leaving.

As I walked back to my desk I thought, "What the hell is the purpose of this agency if it is not to help the people in the quickest possible time?" I was unskilled at looking busy and doing nothing. I had to find a way to fool the VA gods circling in a holding pattern over my head and keep them from becoming displeased.

Since I was a new and unskilled bureaucrat, knowing no other way to upgrade my gaming skills, I started an afternoon self-improvement program. What I would do between each case was to drag out a regulation or manual and study it. Surely, I would win favor with Mr. GS-13 because I would maintain my twenty-five-cases-per-day quota and advance my knowledge of the rules and laws government devised to help veterans.

It was smooth sailing for more than a month, and I thought I was learning the ropes. Then one morning from the back of the room came, "Mr. Roche, my office!" After I arrived, Mr. GS-13 said, "You still don't understand. You must work the whole eight hours doing only twenty-five cases! You don't spend several hours each day reading regulations and manuals. Do I make myself clear Mr. Roche?" "Oh, yes, sir! Mr. GS-13. I will work real hard to fit in and meet your expectations." As I walked back to my desk I thought, "This relationship is headed for the divorce court."

Fall In, Line up, Dress Right Dress

It seemed as if I were put on earth for one purpose only—to become Mr. GS-13's worst nightmare. To explain, the adjudication department was organized to look like a military parade passing in review. The desks, chairs, bookcases, and waste paper baskets were precisely aligned. In the spirit of trying to be part of the team, I made sure my unit was like everyone else's. That was until I was rear-ended in a car accident and suffered severe whiplash from the collision. My doctor wrote to the VA advising that the front end of my desk be elevated at least four inches above floor level. Poor Mr. GS-13! For more than three months, he had to walk past my work area knowing that harmony within the section was broken. The thrill of maintaining a well-organized section was his dream and goal. Every time he passed my work zone, his blood pressure seemed to jump twenty to thirty points as he looked at the one desk that was different. I was starting to feel sorry for the man.

Discrimination Is a No-No!

No sooner was the room back to order with the front of my desk lowered to floor level than some friends and I disrupted the tranquility of the section once again. One of my friends, with whom I served on active duty, was not promoted to the GS-9 level when he transferred into the division. There were about nine of us who started at the same time; all had no experience and came aboard as GS-9s. My friend, however, who was transferred out of the contact division on the first floor, was transferred to Adjudication at his current grade of GS-7. He had the same educational qualifications as all of us and was far more knowledgeable about the technical aspects of the job. As a group, we went to the union representative and complained that management was discriminating against Charlie. Three levels of management were all shook up by the complaint. There were closed-door meetings and all kinds of subsequent meetings to deal with this crisis.

Then, the unbelievable happened! They promoted him to a GS-9 to restore tranquility and stop any bad press in the newspapers if the word got out. Needless to say, I once again managed to notch my way up another step on Mr. GS-13's "watch your step" list.

Finding the Secret of Looking Busy

Meanwhile my friend, who was now a GS-9, clued me in on the way to look busy when you are ready to shut down and go home at two in the afternoon. He suggested taking each file and reviewing it cover to cover. It's an easy trick to look busy and not get in trouble. This was dynamite information and I thought I could soon be off Mr. GS-13's list. Well, guess what? I screwed up again.

Several months later after I mastered the technique of reviewing a file from cover to cover, I came across a claim that had been denied. In the file was the evidence needed to grant the claim. To make matters worse, the veteran was a neighbor of mine. In my innocence, I thought telling Mr. GS-13 and my neighbor about the find would certainly earn me a civilian citation for actions above and beyond the call to duty.

The morning after I found this treasure, I marched in into Mr. GS-13's cubicle and proudly announced I found an error by the rating board that erroneously denied Mr. Smith his compensation benefits. In a voice that echoed through the entire 5th floor (well, that may be a slight over statement), he responded, "You did *what*?" By the tone of his voice, I knew I had stepped in it again. He asked, "Who else knows about this?" "No one, sir, except you and . . . the . . . veteran, who is my neighbor." I had told my neighbor about the find last night. I got another loud "*What*!" Before he could fully recover, I hit him with a quick, "Isn't that our job, sir? To see that veterans get everything they are entitled to?" "Who do think you are, that you can tell a veteran what he or she is entitled to?" he bellowed. "That is not your job. I'm taking this immediately up to the *Director*." (The Director sits on the left hand side of the God of Gods in VA Land.) He is the local representative of the VA's Secretary of the Department of Veterans Affairs. Poor Mr. GS-13! This most heinous act was committed in his section. I remember he paled and said there was going to be "hell to pay for this." On departing he left me with these chilling words: "You have breached an unpublished administrative policy." Man, I was really confused, how can you breach a policy if they never told you about it?

I learned that morning that you do not go back further than the last rating decision when reviewing a file. Some old timers explained this policy to me. It is known as "Top Sheeting" and it had several purposes:

a.   It hastens the flow of cases through the system.
b.   If the claimant doesn't challenge the denial of benefits within one year, the decision stands. To reopen the claim later may be impossible. The VA has created an administrative mine field to discourage any attempt to reopen a claim.
c.   The executive branch of the government and the budgeters who hide in the back rooms of VA Central Office in Washington give each other a thumbs up every time a veteran fails to find a way to reopen his or her claim.

The Time Has Come to File for a Divorce

For nearly three years, I struggled with Mr. GS-13. I finally realized that I did not want to become a Mr. GS-13; therefore, with a happy heart, I said my farewells, feeling like I was the winner because I walked away with a whole briefcase full of knowledge of how the system really works. It was nearly a decade before an opportunity popped up for me to become an advocate. Now I was ready to do battle in their backyard. I finally felt I could help my fellow comrades.

But this isn't the end of the story. My interest in how the VA treated veterans never wilted. Although the faces may change, the "Mr. or Ms. GS-13" will ensure the gates to receiving benefits will always remain tightly controlled. And convincing a rating board member that being held hostage by post-traumatic stress disorder (PTSD) is a serious medical issue is almost an impossible task.

It is impossible, in many cases, to convince a rating board member of the serious-
ness of PTSD when they have no life experiences to relate it to. I wouldn't be sur-
prised if the closest any of these individuals ever came to experiencing a psychological trauma was when they fell off their bicycles at the early age of five and neither
their mothers nor fathers were around to comfort them.

A story recently leaked about a veteran denied service connection for PTSD because he did not serve in Vietnam. He was awarded a non-service connected rating for
PTSD. When the advocate went to the rating board member who denied the claim, the
board member told the advocate to look at his atlas of Vietnam. "Do you see any cities
called Saigon?" asked the board member. "No," was the answer, "but I do see the city
they renamed. It was renamed Ho Chi Minh City when our troops pulled out." "My
atlas makes no mention of this, therefore the decision stands. If he doesn't like it, let
him appeal it," was the board member's last word on the subject. It's completely
conceivable that veterans may battle this issue for the next two to ten years.

Reward Incompetence

The rewards are great for those bureaucrats who do *not* resist the dismantling process.
When he retired from the VA, a former Director of a VA Regional Office was appointed to the position of Executive Director of the Florida State Department of Veterans Services. He, in turn, brought in his number one enforcer. His "yes" shadow
also retired from the VA and was appointed to the second most important position in
the Florida State Department of Veterans Services. The former VA director and adjudication officer were the movers and shakers of one of the worst run regional offices
in the country. Information released by the Department of Veterans Affairs' Board of
Veteran's Appeals identified this regional office as having an almost 80% remanded
or reversed rate! But to the great VA God in Washington, the Secretary of the Department of Veterans Affairs, the Florida director was serving his master well. Millions
upon millions of dollars were never shipped to Florida to support the growing veteran
population.

It is hard to understand how a VA director and adjudication officer, whose leadership earned them an Al Capone reputation, can now, through Harry Potter's wizardry,
be turned into the Elliott Ness protector of veterans' rights. Will this leadership help
the cause of veterans? A real Elliott Ness would organize task forces and go about
righting all the inequities in Florida. To be an advocate, you have to be committed to
challenge the systems. You cannot be a friend of the Governor or Washington's VA
God of Gods and do the job you signed on to do.

ACKNOWLEDGMENTS

First, I wish to acknowledge Sgt. David Raz (a pseudonym) for his valuable contributions by letting me tell his story of frustration and mental stress when dealing with the VA for the past four years. It takes great courage to hang tough when every instinct says to chuck it. It angers me and saddens me that any veteran has to fight so hard for what should have been a slam-dunk request from a government who gave them the problem.

The second thank you goes to Congressman Michael Bilirakis from Florida's Ninth district and his Palm Harbor staff, Sonja and Shirley, for all the great services they have provided Florida veterans. It was their help that made it possible for Sergeant Raz to accumulate evidence and facts from the VA in a timely manner. Congressman Mike, we are going to lose a great champion of veterans' rights in the House of Representatives when you retire next year.

Third, to my wife of more than a half of century, your input helped me "stay the course."

ABBREVIATIONS

A&A	Aid and Attendance
ACR	American College of Radiology
ADJ	Adjudication
AHCRP	Agency for Healthcare Policy and Research
AL	American Legion
ALJ	Administrative Law Judge
AOJ	Agency of Original Jurisdiction
AMA	American Medical Association
AMIE	Automated Medical Information Exchange System
APC	Armored Personnel Carrier
App.	Appeal
BVA	Board of Veterans Appeals
"C"	Claim File Number
CCEP	Comprehensive Clinical Evaluation Program
CDC	Center for Disease Control and Prevention
CFR	*Code of Federal Regulation*
CHAMPUS	Civilian Health and Medical Program United States
CHAMPVA	Civilian Health and Medical Program Veterans Administration
COLA	Cost of Living Adjustment
COMP	Compensation
COPD	Chronic Obstructive Pulmonary Disease
C&P Exam	Compensation and Pension Examination
CSS#	Claim Number using Social Security Number
CAVC	United States Court of Appeals for Veterans Claims
DAV	Disabled American Veterans
DEPS	Did Not Exist Prior to Service
DMZ	Demilitarized Zone
DNA	Defense Nuclear Agency
DOD	Department of Defense
DOS	Date of Separation
DRG	Diagnostic Related Groups
DSC	Direct Service Connection
DSM IV	*Diagnostic and Statistical Manual of Mental Disorders*

DSWA	Defense Special Weapons Agency
DVA	Department of Veterans Affairs (VA)
DVAMC	Department of Veterans Affairs Medical Center (same as VAMC)
EOD	Entrance on Active Duty
EPA	Environmental Protection Agency
EPS	Existed Prior to Service
EVR	Eligibility Verification Report
FR	*Federal Register*
FTCA	Federal Tort Claims Act
FDA	Federal Drug Administration
FOIA	Freedom of Information Act
FTCA	Federal Tort Claims Act
GSW	Gun Shot Wound
HO	Hearing Officer
IB-56	Physician's Guide for Disability Evaluation Examinations
IOM	Institute of Medicine
IU	Individual Unemployability
JAG	Judge Advocate General
KIA	Killed in Action
KIA/BNR	Killed in Action/Body Not Recovered
LOD	Line of Duty Investigation
MIA	Missing in Action
MOAA	Military Officers Association of America
MOS	Military Occupational Specialty
MR	Morning Report
N/A	Not Applicable
NARA	National Archive and Record Administration
NAS	National Academy of Science
NCI	National Cancer Institute
NCPTSD	National Center for PTSD
NCOA	Noncommissioned Officers Association
NOA	Notice of Appeal
NOD	Notice of Disagreement
NPRC	National Personnel Record Center
NRL	National Research Laboratory
NSC	Non-Service-Connected
NTPR	Nuclear Test Personnel Review
OGC	Office of General Counsel
OIG	Office of Inspector General
P&T	Permanent and Total

PCS	Permanent Change Station
PCT	Porphyria Cutanea Tarda
PFC	Private First Class
POW	Prisoner of War
PTSD	Post-Traumatic Stress Disorder
RAD	Released from Active Duty
RO	Regional Office
RPG	Rocket Propelled Grenade
SBA	Survivors Benefit Program
SC	Service Connected
SCP	Specialized Care Program
SMC	Special Monthly Compensation
SMR	Service Medical Records
SOC	Statement of the Case
SSA	Social Security Administration
SSD	Social Security Disability
SSOC	Supplemental Statement of the Case
TDIU	Total Disability due to Individual Unemployability
TDY	Temporary Duty
USA	United States Army
USAF	United States Air Force
USC	United States Code
USCA	United State Code Annotated
USCG	United States Coast Guard
USCMJ	United States Code of Military Justice
USMC	United States Marine Corps
USN	United States Navy
VA	Veterans Administration
VACOVA	Veterans Administration's Central Office, Washington, DC
VABA	Veterans Administration Benefit Administration
VAC	Veterans Administration Clinic
VAE	Veteran Administration Examination
VAF	Veteran Administration Form
VAHA	Veterans Administration Health Administration
VAHAMO	Veteran Administration Health Administration Mammography Office
VAMC	Veteran Administration Medical Center (DVAMC)
VARO	Veterans Administration Regional Office
VEE	Venezuelan Equine Encephalomyelitis
VFW	Veterans of Foreign Wars
VSO	Veteran Service Officer

VVA	Vietnam Veterans of American
WAC	Women's Army Corps
WIA	Wounded in Action
WWI	World War I
WWII	World War II
WWW	World Wide Web

INTRODUCTION

M embers or former members of the U.S. military are more likely than not to have experienced a psychological trauma while in the service. As for police officers, firefighters, and paramedics, the work environment for military service men and women will always be considered extremely hazardous. Unfortunately, tens of thousands of former veterans have been denied service-connected healthcare and compensation for post-traumatic stress disorder (PTSD) because they were unable to make a case for their claim. Such a claim need not be conclusive but must contain enough evidence to satisfy the initial burden.*

If you were a combat infantry trooper or pilot flying off an aircraft carrier or an aircrew member shot down over enemy territory the VA would most likely rule in your favor. Don't assume that your claim will automatically be accepted as service-related, thus granting benefits.

But suppose you were a cook assigned to a marine unit stationed close to the DMZ (Demilitarized Zone) when a surprise attack on your unit's compound occurred late one night. The events you witnessed that night have kept you prisoner in your own body for more than twenty years. Two decades after leaving Vietnam, you file a claim for disabilities associated with PTSD. It is almost 100% certain that, based on your statement alone, your claim for disabilities benefits will be denied. Why? To a senior claims examiner who most likely never served in combat or, for that matter, in the armed forces, would ask, "Who ever heard of a cook engaging in one on one combat with the enemy? And why did his PTSD take twenty years to surface?" Now, you wait. It is nearly a year before the VA letter arrives denying your claim. The letter states: after careful view of the records, we have determined your claim is not valid. What records? This is the question you will ask the examiner to get your foot in the door.

This is a book about the dos and don'ts of filing a claim for PTSD. The last thing you want to do is submit a claim that the VA will deny because it is not well grounded. Here is what you have to look forward to if you do. First, you have to file a Notice of Disagreement (NOD) with the Regional Office that rejected the claim. An NOD must be filed within one year of the denial date. Failure to file on time will greatly complicate future efforts to reopen your claim. Failure to challenge the VA decision will let the VA assume that you are in agreement with their decision. Six to eight months later, the VA will send you a letter known as a Statement of the Case (SOC). The SOC is a summary of how the VA sees the facts and is used to justify why your claim was denied. You might say that it's the "opening statement" by a defendant (the VA) in a civil action suite brought by you (the plaintiff) against the VA. Now claim processors are supposed to cite the factual reasons why your claim was denied. They are required by statute to cite exactly what evidence justified the denial of benefits. Be alert to generic phrases such as "a preponderance of the evidence is against your claim" or "your records are totally silent as to any reference you were a combat infantry soldier." Such statements do not pass the litmus test. Despite the law, maybe one out of ten SOCs will cite the factual evidence which justified the denial of benefits.

Step two, you must respond to the SOC within sixty days, addressing only one issue: why your claim is well grounded. It has been nearly a year since you submitted the original claim. You scratch your head and ask, "What do they mean my PTSD problems didn't start in Vietnam?"

About six to eight months later, the mail carrier delivers another letter from the VA. This time it is called a Supplement Statement of the Case (SSOC). They have rejected your arguments supporting why your claim is valid. You have sixty days to respond. This time you ask to meet with a hearing officer. Again you must wait more than six months before the VA notifies you that a meeting has been scheduled with a hearing officer.

The next letter will tell you that your case is being certified to be forwarded the Board of Veterans' Appeals (BVA). At this point your claim has been in the system nearly three years and you are no closer to obtaining benefits.

Your claim now sits in a locked file until the BVA calls for it to be sent to Washington. Again the magic numbers seem to be six to eight months for action. Once your claim gets to the BVA, another six months may pass before a decision is issued that advises you of the findings.

In total, the time spent with the BVA will add another eighteen months to the process. Here we are, nearly four and half years later, and the only issue so far addressed is whether your claim was valid.

Let's say the BVA agrees with you and remands your case back to the Regional Office of origin. Now the Regional Office will reevaluate the case to determine if the evidence is sufficient to grant service-connection status for your PTSD. Hold on, you're looking at nearly another year before someone gets back to you with that decision.

We are now over the five-year mark, still waiting to see if we will be granted benefits. If the VA does not grant service-connection for your PTSD, the only course is to start all over again with the appeal process. It is at this point many veterans throw up their hands in total frustration and quit trying to receive benefits.

The keys to successfully submitting a winning claim are planning, knowing as much as you can about PTSD, documenting events that caused the psychological trauma, and understanding how the VA thinks. Believe this, they make big-time errors. But this book will help you avoid pitfalls that could result in the rejection of your claim.

Chapter 1 will provide background information necessary to understand the crippling affects of PTSD. Understanding the ABCs of the disorder will help you identify the level of disability you are coping with.

Chapter 2 tells how thousands of VA claims for PTSD more than likely were denied because direct service connection for PTSD was blocked by simply requiring the Bronze Star and the Air Medal when awarded was for heroism. Without a "V" device for these medals, per Operational Manual, M21-1 subchapter 11, section (or §)11.37, a veteran had to prove he or she engaged in direct combat with the enemy and the traumatic event was the direct cause of the PTSD.

Chapter 3 is where you will meet Sgt. David Raz. He is a Vietnam veteran with whom I have worked for nearly four years. It has been an uphill battle all the way, but we still are in the fight. He has granted me permission to tell his story, and show his evidence that is on record. It was extremely hard for him to dig up his past and make his life an open book. His story is no different than the hundreds of thousands of PTSD victims who have tried to deal with the VA and lost. We have managed to storm three-quarters of the way up the mountain. The VA still holds the high ground, but not for long. Read this story before you submit your claim for PTSD so you can plan your strategy.

Chapter 4 opens the door to what the VA adjudication process is supposed to do according to the laws and its regulations when deciding a claim for PTSD. The action word is "supposed." As you will see, what the system is supposed to do and what it does are often quite different.

Chapter 5 introduces you to the basics that you must know before filing a claim. What kind of claim are you going to file? Is it an original claim or perhaps a reopened claim, or is it an informal claim? Not knowing which claim to submit can lead to a deathblow for your benefits.

Chapter 6 explains your responsibility when preparing a claim. Like everything you do in life, there is a right way and a wrong way. Most important, you must file a claim that meets the four critical elements for any claim. If you fail to meet any one of these elements, there is no way you will be granted service connection for PTSD.

Chapter 7 is about the required Compensation and Pension Examination. This is another VA minefield that takes heavy casualties. In Sergeant Raz's story you will come across a document evaluating his PTSD. While he was required to have this examination, it was not performed by a psychiatrist or even by a psychologist. So who is left in the VA medical feeding chain? How about a *nurse practitioner*? As our case rolls to the finish line, it's going to be interesting to see who will prevail in deciding Sergeant Raz's case. Will it be the findings of a board-certified psychiatrist with thirty years' experience or will it be a two-year graduate student majoring in medicine? If it turns out like several of my previous cases, the rating board will base its decision on the findings of the least qualified medical source.

Chapter 8 is devoted to helping veterans qualify for 100% compensation benefits if their level of PTSD prevents them from being employed. The courts ruled that if your PTSD prevents you from earning a living, it does not matter what percentage your disability is rated. In theory it could be as low as 10%.

Chapter 9 is titled "Prove it or Lose It." If your claim is not properly supported by the right kind of evidence, there is no way you can prevail. This chapter is designed to give you a way to find evidence to support your claim. Even though the VA has a duty to assist you in looking for evidence, it would be foolish to depend on them. Only you can provide the energy and interest to submit a winning claim.

Chapter 10 explains how to organize the evidence, assemble your evidence package, and submit it to the VA. There are many kinds of daily experiences on active duty that could cause PTSD. Always remember serving in the military is a 24/7/365 job. Therefore anything that changes your life and affects your ability to adjust to a normal post-service life style is a service-incurred disability. Never forget that within the executive branch of the government there are powerful individuals who are high on slogans but short on support. The purpose of this book is to minimize the chances of your claim being denied for PTSD. If benefits are denied and you do challenge the VA with an appeal, be prepared to hold the course for a period of three to five years. Yes, even ten years. There are no fast-track procedures that would put your appeal ahead of other claims in disputes with the VA. This book will provide you with the means of moving your claim through the process without going the appeal route.

Chapter 11 concerns your rights and how to protect them. It discusses what a well-grounded claim is all about and the consequences for failing to submit a well-documented claim. You will be introduced to precedent-setting decisions by the U.S. Court of Appeals for Veterans Claims that might have an effect on your claim.

Chapter 12 will acquaint you with specific court decisions that are related to PTSD claims. These cases were selected because they represent some of the most difficult claims to be approved.

Notes

* VA's *Duty to Assist Act.*

POST-TRAUMATIC STRESS DISORDER

What Is Post-traumatic Stress Disorder?

Post-traumatic stress disorder (PTSD) is a psychological disorder with a long recorded history of incapacitating hundreds of thousands of individuals who were in combat or traumatized by an event in their lives. It can occur following the experience or witnessing of life-threatening events such as military combat, natural disasters, terrorist incidents, serious accidents, or violent personal assaults. People who suffer from PTSD often relive the experience through nightmares and flashbacks, have difficulty sleeping, and feel detached or estranged. These symptoms can be severe enough and last long enough to significantly impair the person's daily life.

PTSD is marked by clear biological changes as well as psychological symptoms. PTSD is complicated by the fact that it frequently occurs in conjunction with related disorders such as depression, substance abuse, problems of memory and cognition, and other problems of physical and mental health. The disorder is also associated with an impaired ability to function in social or family life, which can manifest itself as occupational instability, marital problems and divorce, family discord, and difficulties in parenting.

Despite popular belief, post-traumatic stress disorder is not a new medical phenomenon that surfaced during the Vietnam War. It has affected warriors for more than twenty-seven hundred years. Neither the victors nor the defeated can escape the horrific after-effects of war. Every person who was ever called to serve or defend his or her country is a possible victim of this disorder.

In 1980 the American Psychiatric Association (APA) published a standard to diagnose traumatized victims who became dysfunctional as a result of their traumatic experience. The *Diagnostic and Statistical Manual of Mental Disorders, 3rd Edition (DSM-III)* wasn't accepted as a standard by the Veterans Administration (VA) Medical Administration for psychiatric service related disability until 1986.[1] The VA now uses the updated fourth edition as its standard. Before the 1986 change of direction, the VA and military doctors commonly diagnosed veterans demonstrating symptoms of PTSD as having a personality disorder, obsessive-compulsive disorder, paranoia, or schizophrenia, but never with PTSD.

By diagnosing individuals with one of these illnesses, the Department of Defense

(DOD) and VA had no lawful duty to compensate these disabled veterans.[2] The law was quite clear: if a veteran had any one of these congenital illnesses, he or she was barred from receiving medical or monetary support. The rational was that congenital medical problems were not the result of serving in the U.S. Armed Forces.

Many of these veterans joined the ranks of the thousands of homeless wanderers. Dysfunctional veterans had a high death rate in automobile accidents and suicides. The genesis for chronic alcoholism and drug addiction is rooted deeply in PTSD.

When considering the hundreds of thousands of individuals who can be ignored by the movers and shakers within an administration their care translates into billions of dollars that can be directed for other purposes. The executive branch of the government—including the White House, the Office of Management and Budget, and the Veteran's Administration—generates billions of dollars in savings annually at the expense of veterans' compensation and health care. The technique is invisible and so does not raise the interest of congressional oversight committees.

Those in the Secretary's Office claim they do not have the necessary computer memory to establish a databank to collect information concerning the number of claims denied annually. How strange it is that an employee could take home the personal data for 26.5 million veterans on a disk and portable hard drive.

Here is an example of how the VA plays the game and what the consequences are for the veteran population: In fiscal years 2003 and 2004, the VA announced that it notified 1,530,000 veterans of their decisions on their claims. Of those who were notified, 330,000 were added to the roll. No explanation was offered concerning the 1,200,000 claims that were not added to the rolls. Let us be conservative and say the VA denied 600,000 claims at an average benefit rate of $500 per month. That would equate to a savings of $7 billion over a two-year period. Veterans with health insurance who seek medical services from the VA Health Administration would have their insurance company charged back for their care. This amount equals hundreds of millions of dollars annually.

If an active duty member is determined to be unfit for worldwide service, he or she must be evaluated by a medical evaluation board. The military uses the VA disability rating schedules to determine the degree of disability for those appearing before their boards. Suppose the air force medical board found an airman 40% disabled because of PTSD. This finding requires that he be medically separated from active service. Military regulations hold that if an individual is to be medically separated and is rated 30% or higher, he or she will be medically retired.

What happens if this person served in WWI, WWII, the Korean War, Vietnam, or during the '60s, '70s, or '80s and has PTSD? Because the VA did not recognize PTSD as an illness prior to 1986, this individual would be separated from the military without medical retirement benefits or assistance from the Department of Veterans Affairs.

The general public's attitude toward people who are mentally ill historically has been extremely intolerant; most would shun them rather than make physical contact.

A good example of this attitude was made public during WWII by an incident caused by Gen. George C. Patton. General Patton was on an inspection tour of an army field hospital when he observed a soldier sitting on a bunk sobbing. He told the soldier to get a hold of himself and behave like a man. The soldier apparently responded with a statement that he was "afraid." The general became so enraged that he grabbed the soldier and struck him while shouting he would "have no cowards" in his army. Patton ordered the hospital commander to send the soldier immediately to the front.

This intolerance demonstrated by General Patton of those handicapped by traumatic incidents often still flows just below the surface in today's military. A career noncommissioned officer (NCO) or officer will try to hide his symptoms so as not to destroy his career, forfeit retirement benefits, or subject himself to unnecessary discrimination owing to lack of knowledge regarding mental health issues.

Another policy generated during the Regan Administration (1981–1989) was the reason why thousand upon thousands of mentally dysfunctional individuals were sent to halfway houses.[3] During 1982, Reagan's administration initiated fiscal changes to reduce the operational cost of running the government. One of these changes was to cut funds for long-term institutional care for the mentally challenged. The reason was simply, "it was more cost effective" to send mentally dysfunctional individuals to halfway houses than to spend the money on their treatment or support. It wasn't too long before funds started to dry up, closing the centers and leaving individuals with no option but to move on to the streets. They became "the walking dead" in every town, city, and state. Many of these individuals were former GIs who served during WWII, Korea, and Vietnam. It was a budget coup for the administration to force local charities to pick up the expense for these homeless people.

During the twentieth century alone, the name for post-traumatic stress disorder was changed three times, but the effects are the same. Doughboys of WWI who succumbed to the psychological traumas of open-trench warfare were identified as suffering from "shell shock." Next, the GI Joes of WWII and Korea who showed the symptoms of psychological trauma were said to have "combat fatigue." Finally, in 1986 combat troops experiencing severe trauma in Vietnam were diagnosed as suffering from PTSD. The American Psychiatric Association added "post-traumatic stress disorder" to the *Diagnostic and Statistical Manual of Mental Disorders, 3rd Edition* in 1980.[4]

However, it was 1986 before the VA considered rating claims for PTSD under the APA standard. Imagine being tagged by the Department of Veterans Affairs as crazy for twenty-seven years. I remember when they started rating PTSD claims. It was in the early 1980s and of those vets granted compensation benefits for PTSD the majority were rated between 0% and 30%. The rating system was devised to compensate a veteran for the loss of their ability to earn a living. A person who has no injuries or illness is said to be 100% whole. A person with PTSD, for example, who is medically diagnosed with definite impairment in the ability to establish or maintain effective and wholesome relationships with people is rated 30% disabled. The earliest VA records available (1986) confirm that this group of veterans comprised 71% of all those on the rolls through 1986. It is truly remarkable that, with all the data available and the advanced collecting software that the VA has not tracked how many claims are received each year and how many claims are denied for any given year. What is known is that of the twenty-five million veterans in the United States, only 10% are on the VA rolls for compensation benefits.

Winning a claim for post-traumatic stress disorder has always been difficult for a veteran. Through the years the VA has arbitrarily rejected thousands of claims based on PTSD disabilities. Sergeant Raz's story, which is explored in chapter 3, is no exaggeration of the difficulty imposed on veterans suffering from this disorder.

VA Marketing of PTSD Information

One of the ways the Department of Veterans Affairs markets its public persona is through a government-identified website for the National Center for Post-traumatic Stress Disorder (NCPTSD).[5] When researching background information for this book, I came across this website by accident. My first thought was this information was being presented by a nongovernment research group. However, suspicion was aroused at the end of the article when the authors stated that it could be used by any one, as it was information in the public domain. Following the links it provided lead me to the NCPTSD home page, which identified itself as a source of information sponsored by the VA. Looking for further information that the NCPTSD was a division of the VA, website I pointed my browser to the Department of Veterans Affairs official home page.[6] The NCPTSD is not mentioned in any of the official hyperlinks associated with the VA website. I did find it when I used their internal search engine. That is not to say that the information is not valid for gaining a basic understanding of this disability.

The National Center for Post-traumatic Stress Disorder was created within the Department of Veterans Affairs in 1989 in response to a congressional mandate to address the needs of veterans with military-related PTSD. Its mission was and remains: "to advance the clinical care and social welfare of America's veterans through research, education, and training in the science, diagnosis, and treatment of PTSD and [other] stress-related disorders."[7] This website is provided as an educational resource concerning PTSD and other enduring consequences of traumatic stress.[8]

Understanding PTSD

PTSD is not new. There are written accounts of similar symptoms that go back to ancient times, and there is clear documentation in the historical medical literature starting with the Civil War, when a PTSD-like mental disability was known as "Da

Costa's Syndrome." There are particularly good descriptions of post-traumatic stress symptoms in the medical literature on combat veterans of World War II and on Holocaust survivors.

Careful research and documentation of PTSD began in earnest after the Vietnam War. The National Vietnam Veterans' Readjustment Study estimated in 1988 that the prevalence of PTSD in that group was 15.2% at that time and that 30% had experienced the disorder at some point since returning from Vietnam.

PTSD has subsequently been observed in all veteran populations that have been studied, including World War II, Korean conflict, and Persian Gulf populations and in United Nations peacekeeping forces deployed to other war zones around the world. There are remarkably similar findings of PTSD in military veterans in other countries. For example, Australian veterans who served in Vietnam experience many of the same symptoms that American veterans experience.

PTSD is not only a problem for veterans, however. There are unique cultural and gender-based aspects of the disorder, and it occurs in men and women, adults and children, Western and non-Western cultural groups, and all socioeconomic strata. A national study of American civilians conducted in 1995 estimated that the lifetime prevalence of PTSD was 5% in men and 10% in women.[9]

How Does PTSD Develop?

Most people who are exposed to a traumatic, stressful event experience some of the symptoms of PTSD in the days and weeks following exposure. Available data suggest that about 8% of men and 20% of women soon develop PTSD, and roughly 30% of these individuals develop a chronic form that persists throughout their lifetimes.[10]

The course of chronic PTSD usually involves periods where symptoms increase followed by periods of remission or decrease, although some individuals may experience symptoms that are unremitting and severe. Some older veterans, who report a lifetime of only mild symptoms, experience significant increases in symptoms following retirement, severe medical illness in themselves or their spouses, or reminders of their military service (such as reunions or media broadcasts of the anniversaries of war events).[11]

How Is PTSD Assessed?

In recent years, a great deal of research has been aimed at developing and testing reliable assessment tools. It is generally thought that the best way to diagnose PTSD— or any psychiatric disorder for that matter—is to combine findings from structured interviews and questionnaires with physiological assessments. A multi-method approach especially helps address concerns that some patients might be either deny-ing or exaggerating their symptoms.

How Common Is PTSD?

An estimated 7.8% of Americans will experience PTSD at some point in their lives, with women (10.4%) twice as likely as men (5%) to develop PTSD. About 3.6% of U.S. adults aged eighteen to fifty-four (5.2 million people) have PTSD during the course of a given year. This represents a small portion of those who have experienced at least one traumatic event; 60.7% of men and 51.2% of women reported at least one traumatic event in their lifetime. The traumatic events for men most often associated with PTSD are rape, combat exposure, childhood neglect, and childhood physical abuse. The most traumatic events for women are rape, sexual molestation, physical attack, being threatened with a weapon, and childhood physical abuse.[12]

About 30% of the men and women who have spent time in war zones experience PTSD. An additional 20% to 25% have had single episodes of PTSD at some point in their lives. More than half of all male Vietnam veterans and almost half of all female Vietnam veterans have experienced "clinically serious stress reaction symptoms." PTSD has also been detected among veterans of the Gulf War, with some estimates running as high as 8%.

Who Is Most Likely to Develop PTSD?

Here are several examples:

- those who experience greater stressor magnitude and intensity, unpre-dictability, uncontrollability, sexual victimization, real or perceived responsi-bility, and betrayal;
- those with preexisting vulnerability factors such as genetics, early age of onset and longer-lasting childhood trauma, lack of functional social support, and concurrent stressful life events;
- those who report greater perceived threat or danger, suffering, upset, terror, and horror or fear; and
- those with a social environment that produces shame, guilt, stigmatization, or self-hatred.

What Are the Consequences Associated with PTSD?

People with PTSD tend to have abnormal levels of key hormones involved in the body's response to stress. Thyroid function also seems to be enhanced in people with

PTSD. Some studies have shown that cortisol levels in those with PTSD are lower than normal and epinephrine and norepinephrine levels are higher than normal. People with PTSD also continue to produce higher than normal levels of natural opiates after the trauma has passed. An important finding is that the neurohormonal changes seen in PTSD are distinct from and actually opposite to those seen in major depression. The distinctive profile associated with PTSD is also seen in individuals who have both PTSD and depression.

PTSD is associated with an increased likelihood of co-occurring psychiatric disorders. In a large-scale study, 88% of men and 79% of women with PTSD met criteria for another psychiatric disorder. The co-occurring disorders most prevalent for men with PTSD were alcohol abuse or dependence (51.9%), major depressive episodes (47.9%), conduct disorders (43.3%), and drug abuse and dependence (34.5%). The disorders most frequently co-morbid with PTSD among women were major depressive disorders (48.5%), simple phobias (29%), social phobias (28.4%), and alcohol abuse or dependence (27.9%.)

Headaches, gastrointestinal complaints, immune system problems, dizziness, chest pain, and discomfort in other parts of the body are common in people with PTSD. Often, medical doctors treat the symptoms without being aware that they stem from PTSD.

How Is PTSD Treated?

PTSD is treated by a variety of forms of psychotherapy and drug therapy. There is no definitive treatment and no cure, but some treatments appear to be quite promising, especially cognitive-behavioral therapy, group therapy, and exposure therapy. Exposure therapy involves having the patient repeatedly relive the frightening experience under controlled conditions to help him or her work through the trauma.

Studies have also shown that medications help ease associated symptoms of depression and anxiety and help with sleep. The most widely used drug treatments for PTSD are selective serotonin reuptake inhibitors, such as Prozac and Zoloft. At present, cognitive-behavioral therapy appears to be somewhat more effective than drug therapy. However, it would be premature to conclude that drug therapy is less effective overall since drug trials for PTSD are at a very early stage. Drug therapy appears to be highly effective for some individuals and is at least somewhat helpful for many more. In addition, recent findings on the biological changes associated with PTSD have spurred new research into drugs that target these biological changes, which may lead to much increased efficacy.

PTSD also significantly affects psychosocial functioning, independent of co-morbid conditions. For instance, VA studies have found that Vietnam veterans with PTSD have profound and pervasive problems in their daily lives. These include problems with family and other interpersonal relationships, problems with employment, and involvement with the criminal justice system.

Let's See What's on the Other Side of the Coin

The above information is revealing and if used as a source for basic insight into PTSD it has its merits. You cannot file a claim based solely on the information in this book. To do so is to invite a denial of benefits. As previously stated, if you go down this road you might never have your claim for PTSD benefits approved.

Complexities in Diagnosing PTSD

PTSD is unusual when compared to other psychiatric conditions. You cannot be diagnosed unless you have met the "stressor criterion," meaning you were exposed to an event that was considered traumatic. Examples of events that meet the stressor criterion are: you were the sole survivor of an aircraft accident or buried alive for several days because an earthquake collapsed the building you were in.

Experienced clinicians will tell us that the symptoms of PTSD vary from one patient to another. Because the psychological makeup of each person differs, differing ability to manage a catastrophic stressful event will result in one person developing PTSD while another individual experiencing the same event will not. This observation also leads to the acceptance that trauma, like pain, cannot be seen externally.

Before a traumatic experience is recognized as a threat, it must be screened through what are known as the cognitive and emotional processes of the mind. It is this individual difference in the appraisal process that produces different traumatic thresholds. That is why some people are more vulnerable to developing clinical symptoms of PTSD after experiencing a traumatic event.

A major problem encountered with PTSD claims is that it is often misdiagnosed. There are many diverse diagnoses that share symptoms with PTSD, includeing anxiety disorder, depressive disorder, organic mental disorder, adjustment disorder, personality disorder, and, in some cases, even psychosis. Clinicians tell us that PTSD is known to coexist with other mental disorders. In order for a rating board member to provide the claimant with the benefits to which he or she are entitled, the board must carefully scrutinize all the medical evidence of record, making certain that they do not prematurely judge the evidence. The danger is great that an inexperienced physician or rating board member will fail to recognize the overlap-ping symptoms common between PTSD and some other forms of neurosis and wrongfully conclude that the claimant does not suffer from PTSD. This is one reason why your supporting medical evidence must be very specific about the symptoms and diagnosis of your condition.

Sex-Related Trauma

Sex-related traumatic events are considered stressors. By direction, rating board members have been told that they must accept the fact that rape, sexual assault, or some other forms of sexual wounding are stressors. Violent events such as these are considered to be stressful incidents by almost anyone. Rating board members are instructed that sexual harassment is also a stressor but much more difficult to corroborate. Still, sexual harassment should never be ruled out as a stressor. Repeated incidences of sexual harassment collectively could turn the victim's life into a living psychological hell. This would qualify as a stressor by acceptable medical standards.

If your claim was denied because the rating board did not consider the trauma associated with sexual harassment as a valid cause of your PTSD, the denial should be challenged. VA policy in recent years has put rating board members on notice that when rating sexual traumatic claims, they must not display any form of moral judgment. The fact that a person is sexually active in no way diminishes the trauma of some form of sexual assault.

Coexisting Psychiatric Disorders

By decisions of the U.S. Court of Appeals for Veterans Claims and the medical community at large, the VA has accepted the fact that it is possible for PTSD to actively coexist with another psychiatric disorder. However, that does not mean that individual rating board members grasp or rate PTSD claims with a thorough understanding of this acceptable medical standard. *Always remember that rating board members do not have a formal education or experience in the complexities of medicine or law.* What they do have is a manual, a regulation, some in-house guidance from the adjudication officer, an extremely heavy caseload, and a great deal of discretionary power. My experience has been that if they are going to err they do so in favor of the government. This means if they don't understand the medical or legal aspects of the claim, they will simply deny it and allow the veteran try to argue it out through the appeal process.

Some Fundamental Facts about PTSD

PTSD is not a psychosis. It is a neurosis and, as such, the patient will not share those symptoms common of a patient suffering from a psychosis. In order for a physician to diagnose a neurosis, the symptoms must fit into a group of symptoms common to that condition. If the patient does not demonstrate those required symptoms associated with the condition, the doctor will not diagnose the veteran as having a neurosis. The presence of cognitive disorders is not a symptom of PTSD. However, a PTSD patient may experience flashbacks—a form of visual hallucination that is very detailed and relates directly to the stressful event.

PTSD can occur at anytime during your lifetime. However, VA policy is if an individual is diagnosed with "partial PTSD" or with "PTSD features," he or she is not considered to have PTSD for compensation purposes.

Secondary Service-connected Disorders

The VA does recognize that there can be a relationship between chronic PTSD and substance abuse. This policy decision, made in the early 1990s, was not endorsed by the executive branch of the government. It was the U.S. Court of Appeals for the Federal Circuit that forced the VA to consider this issue. Alcohol and drug abuse per se cannot be rated or granted a service-connected disability status. This designation is specifically barred by law because it is considered an action of willful misconduct. However, there have been many hotly debated appeals before the U.S. Court of Appeals for Veterans Claims. The frequency of this issue before the court, in addition to PTSD appeals, demonstrates the doggedness the VA rating boards demonstrate in holding the line on PTSD claims.

When substance abuse is the consequences of some other medical condition, it can be considered secondary to the primary medical problem and thus recognized as service connected. Substance abuse (alcohol or drug) can coexist with PTSD just as other forms of neurosis or psychoses can co-exist with PTSD. It is not unusual for multiple disorders to exist simultaneously and have no clinical relationship to each other. Because of the uniqueness of this possible relationship, you should make certain that your medical examiners clearly define the relationship between alcohol and drug abuse and the service-connected PTSD in their claim statements.

Alcohol or substance abuse can quickly complicate what otherwise appears to be a clear-cut case of a service-related PTSD. The claimant must make certain that his or her physician clearly states that the current drug or alcohol condition is secondary to, a symptom of, or caused by PTSD. If this fact is not plainly made in the medical assessment by your physician, you can bet the claim will be denied. The VA will not accept a simple diagnosis of this relationship. The medical evidence furnished by your physician must support the diagnosis of a secondary relationship between alcohol or substance abuse and PTSD.

If secondary service-connected status is granted for alcohol or drugs, it will be considered part of the primary disorder and, as such, no additional compensation will be authorized. However, if subsequently, the substance abuse condition is responsible for triggering another medical condition such as cirrhosis of the liver, this condition would be rated as service-connected and compensation would be in order for the liver problem.

Chapter 1: What Have We Learned?

The standard medical manual used by VA to rate a claim for PTSD is *Diagnostic and Statistical Manual of Mental Disorders, 4th Edition*. The manual's definition of PTSD is at http://allpsych.com/disorders/dsm.html. If you do not have access to a computer, your local library should have a copy of the manual in their reference section.

We will never know how many PTSD claims are denied each year until the VA is required to obtain from their regional offices a monthly accounting of how many veterans have applied for PTSD benefits. If there are twenty-five million veterans living, from WWII through Gulf War II, the VA's 10% disabled figure is extremely skewed to the right. There has been a drastically increase number of veterans granted PTSD since the courts and Congress increased their oversight in 1989.

Notes

1. American Psychiatric Association (APA), "309.89 Post-traumatic Stress Disorder," in *Diagnostic and Statistical Manual of Mental Disorders: DSM-IV-R, 4th ed. revised.* (Washington, DC: American Psychiatric Association, 2000), http://www.cirp.org/library/psych/ptsd/.
2. Principals Relating to Service Connection, 38 CFR 3.304(c), March 7, 2002.
3. Ann Palmer, "20th Century History of the Treatment of Mental Illness: A Review," http://www.mentalhealthworld.org/29ap.html.
4. APA, *DSM-IV*.
5. National Center for Post-Traumatic Stress Disorder, http://www.ncptsd.va.gov/.
6. Department of Veterans Affairs, http://www.va.gov.
7. National Center for Post-Traumatic Stress Disorder, http://www.ncptsd. va.gov/.
8. Yancy v. Principi, Docket Number 01-298, CAVC, April 27, 2004.
9. Palmer, "20th Century History of the Treatment of Mental Illness."
10. APA, *DSM-IV*.
11. Palmer, "20th Century History of the Treatment of Mental Illness."
12. Ibid.

2 | TWO LITTLE WORDS

In chapter 3, I will introduce you to Sgt. David Raz and his five-year struggle for benefits resulting from PTSD. You will see how he became a victim of the Veterans Administration's game of *deny, deny, and deny* that has been in play for decades. Why would the VA do this? I can only guess that administrators do not want to be forced into budget increases year after year. This position is supported by a speech made in the House of Representatives.

Congressman Lane Evens Musters Support for Vets

The ranking democratic member of the Budget Resolution for Fiscal Year 2005 Conference Committee, Representative Lane Evens, made this statement before the House on May 19, 2004. His speech was to encourage members on both sides of the House to vote against the concurrent resolution laying out the congressional budget for the U.S. Government for fiscal year 2005.

> Mr. Chairman, I rise in opposition to S. Con. Res. 95. As too many of us in this body know, this budget is a sham. It fails to account for the real costs of waging the war in Iraq and Afghanistan. At least on the House side, it allows tax cuts for the wealthiest Americans to go forward unchecked, while spending for important domestic programs is laid to waste.
>
> Among those high priorities that will be *severely under funded is veterans' health care*. Committee on Veterans Affairs Chairman Christopher H. Smith and I submitted Views and Estimates to the Budget Committee requesting that it add $2.5 billion to VA's budget for fiscal year 2004. This was not a "pie in the sky" request, but rather, focused on maintaining current services, restoring funds from the Administration's failed proposals to increase co-payments and introduce new enrollment fees, and slightly enhancing some services that will have to respond to the needs of demobilizing troops. The resolution we are voting on today will make less than half of these funds available to VA's discretionary programs.
>
> Mr. Chairman, sadly, I realize VA programs are among those considered "protected" in this budget fiasco. Many social programs will fare worse. Unfortunately, that's not good enough for our veterans, especially during a time of war

when we should be most sensitive toward keeping our promises to the men and women who have borne the battle.

Many of the major veterans' organizations have expressed great concern about the budget. As under funded as the budget was by the Committee's reckoning, it is even more so according to the Independent Budget. The four major veterans service organizations who prepare this document estimate that VA requires almost $4 billion to maintain its services in fiscal year 2005. And that's not the worst of it— budget process bills that may be put forth in the near future may use the projections of future years spending to bind us to even more inadequate budgets. So as bad as fiscal year 2005 looks, the outlook for future years could be even bleaker. Mr. Chairman, we must do better by the veterans who have served us. We must do better by the American people. Vote NO on accepting this Conference Report.

The VA Flow Chart

The management level decision to adopt only a portion of the prerequisites for awarding the Bronze Star[1] was greatly influenced by this type of budget posturing. Adding two words—"V" device—to the statutory requirements for the Air Medal[2] slammed the door on many PTSD claims. Thousands of Vietnam and Gulf War veterans failed to qualify for direct service connection for PTSD because their awards were not considered "conclusive evidence." These administrative changes had an enormous impact on how PTSD claims are processed. All the key rules governing PTSD claims are discussed in chapter 4.

Had the St. Petersburg Regional Office followed the law as Congress approved it, Sergeant Raz's claim for PTSD should have been resolved in six to eight months in his favor. The VA claimed his PTSD did not qualify for direct service connection since his Bronze Star had no "V" (for Valor) device. As you read chapter 3 you will see how the VA used various bureaucratic and administrative techniques to sabotage Sergeant Raz's will to hold the course.

It is important to know what your rights are and what the VA can and cannot do. When filing a claim do not expect the VA to do the legwork to develop the evidence necessary to establish your claim. They are directed to assist you by statutes, regulations caselaw, and their own manuals. However, to be uninformed of the claiming process is to invite a denial of the benefits. When filing a claim for PTSD, know the rules better than the adjudicators.

It is the Congress who authorizes all agencies of the government to execute their duties in accordance with the statutes they pass. The laws governing the Department of Veterans Affairs are marshaled under *Title 38 U.S. Code*, section 38 of the *Code of Federal Regulations*, general counsel opinions, and decisions rendered by the

U.S. Court of Appeals for Veterans Claims and the U.S. Court of Appeals for the Federal Circuit.

Title 38 U.S. Code

Chapter 11, section 1154 of *Title 38* authorizes assistance to veterans who are injured, traumatized, or disabled by disease on or after January 1, 1947. Sub-paragraph (b) specifically addresses the needs of veterans suffering from PTSD.

When reading chapter 4, take note there is no mentioning of a narrow or restrictive guideline pertaining to presumptive of service–connection tied to combat with the enemy. The bottom line of section (b) is: *The VA shall accept as sufficient proof of service-connection any disease or injury allegedly incurred in or aggravated during active service. Lay or other evidence will be accepted if such injury or disease is consistent with the circumstances, conditions, or hardships of such service.*

This section also states if the claim is denied, adjudicators must spell out in detail exactly what evidence topples the scales in their favor. The U.S. Court of Appeals for Veterans Claims (CAVC) has said numerous times, "No, No, No, you [the VA] cannot simply say a preponderance of evidence is against the claim." Should you receive such an explanation for the denial of your claim, *appeal it immediately.*

Federal Register Final Notice 06-18-99

As you read through the Federal Register ("Final Notice of Change"), the major amendment that impacted 38 *CFR (Code of Federal Regulations)* §3.304(f) was the removal of references to service department evidence of combat or receipt of specific combat citations. These combat awards, such as the Purple Heart, Combat Infantryman Badge, or similar combat citations were conclusive evidence of the claimed in-service stressor. This changed the procedure a veteran diagnosed with PTSD must follow before service-connection could be granted.

Although this revision is touted as being a more liberal interpretation of 38 CFR §3.304(f), quite the opposite is true. This revision states "if evidence establishes that the veteran engaged in combat," direct service connection will be approved. The questions that must be ask are: What kind of evidence will satisfy this regulatory requirement? Where do I find it? How do I get it? If you can't answer "I know" to each question, you lose. Claim denied!

Each of the three revised paragraphs has one common denominator. Paragraphs one and two declare that the veteran's lay testimony alone *may* establish the occurrence of the claimed in-service stressor. Paragraph three states evidence from sources other than the veteran's service records *may* corroborate the veteran's account of the stressor incident.

The use of the word "may" is an open invitation for adjudicators to say "your statement isn't sufficient to warrant direct service connection; please provide us with details and proof of the traumatic event you're alleging is the reason for your PTSD." Because the VA has not accepted your initial application for PTSD benefits, you are now destined for a lengthy process. This is where adjudicators start telling you they need detailed information confirming the event you are alleging as the cause of your PTSD.

Remember, rating board members are not professionally trained to deal with complex medical or legal issues. They rely on a sort of checklist of questions that is intended to lead them to a proper decision. Their method of resolving decisions is best described as a "Yes or No" guideline of questions. A question is asked; if the answer is "yes," you will do this, if answer is "no," you will do that. Thus by answering all the questions, the rating board members are supposed to arrive at the correct solution.

The easiest way for them to avoid making an error when granting direct service connection is to simply declare the veteran's statement is not sufficient to support service occurrence of the claimed in-service stressor. This way they don't present themselves to management as reckless cowboys letting the steers out of the coral. If they error in favor of the government, their annual merit pay increase is never in jeopardy.

As you read Sergeant Raz's journal, you will see how the St. Petersburg Regional Office avoided concrete decisions for four years and counting. We had to furnish endless reams of paper detailing his traumatic experiences along with medical evaluations by his psychiatrist. With all that, it was necessary to challenge them two times with the appeal process before they relented and granted the benefits. And as you will see, we must now appeal the denial of his claim for Total Disability based on Individual Unemployability (TDIU).

To deny Sergeant Raz's claim for TDIU benefits and deliberately ignore statutes, regulation, general counsel opinions, caselaw and, most importantly, evidence that substantiates his claim, is unbelievable. I don't wish to offend any readers, but I have to say the St. Petersburg Regional Office has a giant set of "brass b——." Their denial letter and our response will be covered in chapter 3.

VA Manual M21-1

VA Manual M21-1 is a detailed procedure manual instructing rating board members and claims examiners what is required when evaluating a claim. Subchapter 11, §11.37 specifically outlines the standards to rate a PTSD claims. Unfortunately, I do not have access to an archive that would trace the flip-flop revision of this particular chapter going back to the 1980s. However, between court cases, revisions to *Title 38 U. S. Code*, and 38 *CFR* §3.3.304(f), the manual seems to indicate that the Veterans Benefits Administration is once again forced to comply with the intent of Congress.

VA Manual M21-1 §11.37 was last revised on March 10, 2004 and reads as follows:

(I) Conclusive Evidence.

a. Any evidence available from the service department indicating that the veteran served in the area in which the stressful event is alleged to have occurred and any evidence supporting the description of the event are to be made part of the record. Corroborating evidence of a stressor is not restricted to service records, but may be obtained from other sources (see *Doran v. Brown,* 6 Vet. App. 283 [1994]). If the claimed stressor is related to combat, in the absence of information to the contrary, receipt of any of the following individual decorations will be considered evidence that the veteran engaged in combat:

- Air Force Cross
- *Air Medal with "V" Device* [italics added]
- Army Commendation Medal with "V' Device
- *Bronze Star Medal with "V" Device* [italics added]
- Combat Action Ribbon
- Combat Infantryman Badge
- Combat Medical Badge
- Combat Aircrew Insignia
- Distinguished Flying Cross
- Distinguished Service Cross
- Joint Service Commendation Medal with "V" Device
- Medal of Honor
- Navy Commendation Medal with "V" Device
- Navy Cross
- Purple Heart
- Silver Star.

Other supportive evidence includes, but is not limited to, plane crash, ship sinking, explosion, rape or assault, duty on a bum ward or in graves registration unit. POW status that satisfies the requirements of 38 CFR 3.1(y) will also be considered conclusive evidence of an in-service stressor.

(2) Personal Assault

Evidence of Personal Assault Personal assault is an event of human design that threatens or inflicts harm. Examples of this are physical assault, domestic battering, robbery, mugging, and stalking.

a. Alternative Evidence. If the military record contains no documentation that a personal assault occurred, alternative evidence might still establish an in-service stressful incident. Examples of such evidence include, (but are not limited to):

◆   records from law enforcement authorities;
◆   records from rape crisis centers, hospitals, or physicians;
◆   pregnancy tests or tests for sexually transmitted diseases; and
◆   statements from family members, roommates, fellow service members, or clergy.

Changing the Meaning of 32 CFR §578.11&12

The Veterans Benefit Administration is being forced to flip flop once again concerning "conclusive evidence" and "direct service connection." Note the requirements set forth for the Bronze Star and Air Medal in this revised change to M21-1 Subchapter 11, §11.35. The VA states for these two medals to qualify as conclusive evidence they must include a "V" device for heroism. But, by doing so, they eliminated several million Vietnam and Persian Gulf veterans from being eligible for direct service connection. Every one of these vets will have to do it the hard way just like Sergeant Raz. But before we declare ourselves defeated, let's look into the Department of Defense's Award Division regulation and see what is necessary to qualify for either one of these awards.

Air Medal
§578.12 Air Medal
a. Criteria. The Air Medal, established by Executive Order on May 11, 1942, is awarded to any person who, while serving in any capacity in or with the army of the United States, has distinguished himself or herself by meritorious achievement while participating in aerial flight. (Fig. 1). Awards may be made to recognize single acts of merit or *sustained operational activities against an armed enemy.* (Italics added.)The required achievement, while of lesser degree than that required for the award of the Distinguished Flying Cross, must nevertheless have been accomplished with distinction above and beyond that normally expected.
578.11 Bronze Star Medal.
a. Criteria. The Bronze Star Medal, established by Executive Order on February 4, 1944, is awarded to any person who, while serving in any capacity in or with the army of the United States, on or after December 7, 1941 shall have distinguished himself or herself by heroic *or meritorious achievement or service not involving participating in aerial flight in connection with military operations against an armed enemy.* (Italics added.)
    (1) Heroism. Awards may be made for *acts* of heroism performed in actual ground combat against an armed enemy which are of lesser degree than required

for the award of the Silver Star.

(2) Meritorious *achievement and service.* Awards may be made to recognize single acts of merit and meritorious service. The required achievement or service, while of lesser degree than that required for the award of the Legion of Merit, must nevertheless have been meritorious and accomplished with distinction.

While reading the official policy concerning the issuance of the Air Medal, did you see where the executive order specifically stated that this decoration would be awarded for heroism? My personal experience during the Korean War earned me an Air Medal for bombing targets deep in North Korea. I assure you the North Koreans were not lighting up the sky with fireworks in celebration of our heroic northward run to targets just south of the Chinese border. Every crewmember of the 98th Bomb Wing earned an Air Medal when he flew ten or more combat missions north of the DMZ.

Now for a few words concerning the VA position on the Bronze Star. Yes! Executive order originating the award states it can be awarded for heroism. But it also states that it can be awarded for meritorious achievement or *service in connection with military operations against an armed enemy.*

The question that comes to mind is how could the Under Secretary for Veterans Benefit Administration overlook such an important criterion that is built into the 32 CFR §578.11? Just think of the hundreds of thousands of soldiers who for one whole year chased "Charlie" up and down the Vietnam peninsula. They would spend endless days away from base camp tracking the enemy; it was the norm to sleep in the mud or wade through snake- and tiger-infested jungles and swamps. However, to all the bureaucrats waging a major attack on vast backlogs of claims action in their citadel accommodations in the center of any city USA, these actions by the ground forces are not considered special achievements.

Chapter 2: What Have We Learned?

1. When the VA adjudicators grant a benefit or denies it, they must give a full explanation of what evidence was used to approve or refuse the claim. Failure to do this is grounds for appeal.

2. It is Congress's intent to make the burden of proving your claim as liberal as possible. As you have seen, the VA will go to extremes to deny benefits.

3. Your word is your bond as demonstrated by the legislation passed by the Congress. However, just because Congress wants to make it easy for you to have your claim processed with as little hassle as possible, it does not mean the VA shares this same commitment to those who serve.

4. Changes that control how the Department of Veterans Affairs operates come

from six sources. They are statutes, regulations, general counsel opinions, inspectors general's staff, caselaw, and acknowledgeable claimants.

5. Look for trigger words in any governing document, or award letters that give a different meaning to Congress's intent, such as using "may" instead of "shall," or adding a word to a regulation that changes its meaning.

6. Do not give up in frustration; if you fail to get what you are claiming and have the proof to support your claim, remember: *appeal, appeal, appeal.*

7. The VA will force a veteran needlessly to search for additional evidence when there is sufficient evidence of record to make a determination.

8. When rating a combat injury or other conditions that obviously had their inception in the service, the rating process is suppose to go forward pending receipt of active duty medical records and all service records.

9. If an injury or medical condition is tied to combat, the veteran's word is sufficient proof of service connection if the circumstance matches the conditions even though there is no proof of the traumatic event.

10. PTSD requires medical evidence that the veteran is currently disabled by PTSD and the disorder is associated with events related to his or her combat experiences.

Notes

1. 32 CFR §578.11, February 4, 1944.
2. 32 CFR §578.12, September 11, 1942.

3 | SGT. DAVID RAZ'S FIVE-YEAR STRUGGLE

Have you ever wondered what it would be like to be so traumatized by serving your country that you could barely function in the civilian world after leaving the service? I've known such men and it really grinds me to see how they are jerked around by an agency chartered to help them. This chapter is in six parts and will acquaint you with an ongoing account of the typical, unnecessary stress veterans claiming PTSD experience when they attempt to collect benefits. This chapter will provide you with techniques to counter the VA's line of attack in denying benefits.

To give you a realistic insight into the claims process and an appreciation for the burden of evidence PTSD victims bear, I'm going to tell you the story of Sgt. David Raz. To protect the real David Raz, others who played a role in helping him, and those who gave their lives for their country, names and places have been changed. But, believe me, the events that unfold are very real. Who knows, this might be your story.

This is Sgt. David Raz's story, told in a journal format. It is put together as a time line, starting when he first applied for PTSD benefits in 2001. His four-year battle with the VA is far from over. In pursuit for PTSD benefits, he was forced to provide evidence that, by law, should not have been required. David was the recipient of the Bronze Star and Purple Heart, which entitles him to direct service connection. However, that is not how the St. Petersburg Regional Office saw it.

Sergeant Raz's campaign to win benefits has been a terrible stressor for a man who is already stressed to the limits. The demand for evidence required resourcefulness and perseverance beyond belief. The last thing the government should do to a man or woman traumatized by war is to force them to stand exposed and dance to the tunes of the bureaucrats. Writing down traumatic and painful memories for others to read is an impossible task for thousands of veterans. Many simply say, "The hell with it! Let the VA get what they can and let the chips fall where they may." A letter denying benefits is the VA's way of saying, "Nice working with you, but good-bye" In David's case, dealing with the VA on a letter-by-letter basis for four years nearly forced him to throw up his hands and quit. There are tens of thousands of David Razes who experienced similar treatment by the VA and did quit.

I have been working with David since February 2001. To date he still hasn't been granted all the entitlements the law provides. However, we have forced the VA to reverse its decision two times, which resulted in establishing service connection for PTSD at the 70% rate.

Sgt. David Raz, sixty-one, was inducted into the army at the age of twenty-six. He was encouraged to apply for VA compensation benefits by his psychiatrist, Dr. Henry Jones. Dr. Jones, a former VA psychiatrist, knew only too well the tortuous existence of the bloodless wounded.

Just before I started working with Sergeant Raz, he filed a claim for PTSD. He told the VA he wanted to reopen his claim. The VA had his records and knew he had shell fragment wounds. He was awarded the Purple Heart because of these injuries. The VA rated him 0% on December 20, 1970, for "shell fragment wound scars right upper eyelid and left scalp."

In *Proscelle v. Derwinski* the court noted that in order to trigger the VA's duty assist, the claimant's evidentiary burden is to submit *sufficient evidence to justify a belief by a fair and impartial individual that the claim is well grounded.* In this case the VA denied his request for increased benefits on the basis his claim for PTSD was not well grounded. However, in similar cases the court has held that the claim was plausible and capable of substantiation.

Part I: 2001[1]

FEBRUARY 28, 2001: VETERAN FILES CLAIM FOR PTSD
Figure 3.1 is David Raz's letter claiming benefits for PTSD.[2] Unknowingly, David used the phrase "reopen my claim." What David did not know was "reopen my claim" implies a previous claim for PTSD was denied. This was not the case. He had no way of knowing that the correct phrase should have been "amend my original claim to include PTSD."

	Fig. 3.1

909 Spruce Drive
Tampa, FL 33756-4033

Department of Veteran Affairs Regional Office
P.O. Box 1437
St. Petersburg, FL 34703-1212

February 28, 2001

Re: CXX-XXX-889
To Whom It May Concern:

I wish to reopen my claim and amend it to include Post Traumatic Stress Disorder.
My file number is CXX-XXX-889. I will be sending documentation at a later date.

Sincerely,

David Raz

MARCH 30, 2001: DOCTOR RELEASES VETERAN
TO RETURN TO WORK

Dr. Henry Jones, David's psychiatrist, sent a letter to Suncoast District Occupational Health Services Office concerning the effects of PTSD as they related to the veteran's work. After six extensive weeks of psychiatric therapy, David was ready to return to work at the U.S. Postal Service. Figure 3.2 shows a copy of Dr. Jones's March 30, 2001, letter to the post office.

| ADULT AND ADOLESCENT PSYCHIATRY
FORENSIC PSYCHIATRY AND HYPNOTHERAPY | Page 1 | **Fig. 3.2** |

HENRY JONES. M.D., P.A.
1234 ROAD EAST, SUITE 1301
CLEARWATER, FL 33750

March 30, 2001

USPS Sun Coast District
Occupational Health Services
P.O. Box 55555
Tampa. FL 33630

Attn: W. Worth, R.N.
RE: David Raz
SS# XXX-XX-7777

Dear Ms. Worth:

I have been treating David Raz since March 25, 1997 for the following conditions:

308.3 —Acute Posttraumatic Stress Disorder
309.81— Chronic Posttraumatic Stress Disorder
309.1— Depressive Reaction Prolonged

On February 9, 2001 he was seen in my office on an emergency basis. He was suffering from an exacerbation of his condition and was unable to work. I had been seeing this patient weekly since than. His last office visit with me was on March 29, 2001 and I feel that he is ready to return to work.

I feel that he is not a risk to himself or to others and he is able to perform the following functions without experiencing a disabling reaction:

* Cope with flexible scheduling.
* Be punctual and demonstrate regular attendance without frequent or extended absenteeism.
* Interact directly and frequently with a variety of coworkers.
* Adapt to limits and standards, and respond appropriately to supervision.
* Handle disagreements with others without exhibiting disruptive behavior in the workplace, for example crying, yelling, threatening, or violent behavior.

* Cope with time constraints and demands. Possess sufficient concentration, *memory* and persistence to perform relatively simple and routine tasks while maintaining a moderate pace of work.
* Make independent decisions and initiate timely action, maintaining concentration and completing complex tasks rapidly.
* Perform job tasks in an effective manner after having received constructive feedback regarding unacceptable job performance.

I certify that David Raz is able to perform the above functions and the job requirements of his position without causing an exacerbation to his condition at present. In addition, I see no activity that this individual cannot presently perform or one that is likely to cause an exacerbation of his condition. This patient has relayed to me that he feels much relieved and that many of the symptoms that occurred at his time exacerbation are no longer present.

I would also like to note that I am speaking strictly from a psychiatric standpoint. Mr. Raz is being followed by Dr. Charles E. Brown M.D., Orthopedic Associates of West Florida, P.A. I have received documentation showing the following diagnosis: Cervical Disc Disease C5—C6 and Degenerative Joint Disease SC Joint Right Shoulder. The patient reports that he is asymptomatic at this time.

If you need any further information, please do not hesitate to communicate with me.

Sincerely,

Henry Jones
Henry Jones, M.D.

AUGUST 24, 2001: VA REQUESTS ADDITIONAL EVIDENCE

The VA sent the letter in figure 3.3, dated August 24, 2001, to the veteran stating they needed additional information before deciding his case. This type of letter is only appropriate when a noncombatant is claiming PTSD. In David's case, the request for this information was totally without merit.

Sending this letter was one of the first errors team 70B made when adjudicating Mr. Raz's claim for PTSD benefits. The VA manual M21-1 states that when a combat veteran is awarded the Purple Heart or Bronze Star, Air Medal with a "V" device, or any one of the other thirteen awards, this is conclusive evidence that the veteran was involved in combat with the enemy. Mind you, shortly after he was discharged in 1970, the VA rated David 0% for shrapnel wounds to the head. Team 70 had this information when they decided that he did not qualify for direct service connection base on conclusive evidence of combat with the enemy. When the records show the veteran was wounded by the enemy, the VA is not to delay the rating process by demanding additional information related to his combat experiences. This is an appealable error that demonstrates the rater was not very knowledgeable about the rules and regulations governing PTSD claims. This is the second letter David received.

Fig. 3.3

COPIED FROM CLAIMS FOLDER DEPARTMENT OF VETERANS' AFFAIRS (317)
DEPARTMENT OF VETERANS AFFAIRS
St. Petersburg Regional Office
P.O. BOX 1437
St. Petersburg, FL 33731

To: David Raz
909 Spruce Drive
Tampa, FL 34703

In Reply Refer 317/VSC/TEAM70/B
C XX-XXX-889

Dear Mr. Raz:

We recently received your application for service-connected benefits on March 1, 2001.

Your VA file number is XX XXX 887. Please have this number available when contacting this office. Your claim will be handled by Team 70. We want you to know that we will help you get evidence to support your recent claim for benefits. Specifically, we are referring to your claim for your post traumatic stress disorder. In this letter we will tell you what evidence is necessary to establish entitlement, what information or evidence we still need from you, and what you can do to help with your claim. It will also tell you when and where to send the information or evidence, what has been done to help with your claim, and who to call if you have questions or need assistance.

VA's Duty to Notify You about Your Claim

The law requires us to explain to you what information or evidence we need to grant the benefit you want. We will tell you when medical evidence is required. Medical evidence includes such things as doctors' records, medical diagnoses, and medical opinions.

We will tell you what necessary information or evidence you must give us, such as income information, or the names and addresses of doctors who treated the veteran's medical condition. We will also tell you what necessary information or evidence we will try to get for you.

VA's Duty to Assist You Obtain Evidence for Your Claim

The law states that we must make reasonable efforts to help you get evidence necessary to support your claim. We will try to help you get such things as medical records, employment records, or records from other Federal agencies. You must give us enough information about these records so that we can request them from the person or agency who has them. It's still your responsibility to make sure these records are received by us.

We will also assist you by providing a medical examination or getting a medical opinion if we decide it's necessary to make a decision on your claim.

If you do not know of any additional evidence you wish us to consider please tell us so in writing, using the enclosed Statement in Support of Claim (VA Form 21-4138).

What Must the Evidence Show to Establish Entitlement?

To establish entitlement for service connected compensation benefits, the evidence must show three things:

- *An injury in military service or a disease that began in or was made worse during military service, or an event in service causing injury or disease.* If we do not yet have them, we will get service medical records and will review them to see if they show you had an injury or disease in service. We will also get other military service records if they are necessary.

OR

- For certain conditions, you don't have to show that you had an injury or disease in service. These are called "presumptive conditions." These are medical conditions that were first shown after service, not during service. For most of these conditions, the evidence must show that you were diagnosed with the condition within one year after you left military service. Longer time limits apply for certain other medical conditions.
- *A current physical or mental disability.* This can be shown by medical evidence or other evidence showing you have persistent or recurrent symptoms of disability. We will get any VA medical records or other medical treatment records you tell us about. If necessary, we may schedule a VA examination for you to get this evidence. You may also submit your own statements or statements from other people describing your physical or mental disability symptoms. We will review this evidence to see if it shows you have a current disability or symptoms of a disability.
- *A relationship between your current disability and an* injury, disease, or event in service. This is usually shown by medical records or medical opinions. We will request this medical evidence for you if you tell us about it. If appropriate, we may also try to get this evidence for you by requesting a medical opinion from a VA doctor, or you can give us a medical opinion from your own doctor.

AUGUST 24, 2001: VA SENDS SECOND LETTER REQUESTING MORE EVIDENCE

This is the second letter dated August 24, 2001. The first one basically said, "Hi! I'm your new buddy. Here is what I can do to help you." The second one states, "If you want to be service-connected for PTSD, you had better get us the following information." In thinking about the letters, it looks like the right hand of team 70 doesn't know what the left hand is doing.

This is a good time to give you a sidebar note of interest. The VA published a fact sheet in December 2004 proudly touting statically data that should make you want to stand up and shout. In the year 2003, the fifty-seven Regional Offices notified 827,000 veterans of decisions concerning their disability claims. According to the VA, 256,000 veterans were added to Compensation and Pension rolls in 2003. If a third grade math class was asked how many veterans were turned down, their answer would be 571,000. So, what are the odds of having a claim approved? You could say seven of ten veterans were denied or, if you prefer, you could say three out of ten were approved. This is why I have said several times: *you have to know the territory.*

SEPTEMBER 13, 2001: VETERAN PUTS THE VA ON NOTICE ABOUT THE CLAIM DATE

Figure 3.4 is an example of a form to be used when the VA does not respond correctly to your intent. David filed VA Form 21-4138 (which can be downloaded from the VA website) restating the intent of his February 28, 2001, letter. His statement stressed that his February 28, 2001, letter was meant to be an "informal claim." If we hadn't filed a statement, the VA would have rated the claim in sixty days. There was no question that team 70 was going to deny the benefit. This action put us back in the game. No matter how they responded, by filing this form we established grounds for appealing that action.

Fig. 3.4

0MB Approved No. 2900-0075 Respondent Burden: 15 minutes

Department of Veterans Affairs   STATEMENT IN SUPPORT OF CLAIM

PRIVACY ACT INFORMATION: The law authorizes us to request the information we are asking you to provide on this form (38 U.S.C. 501(a)) and (b)). The responses you submit are considered confidential (38 U.S.C. 5701). They may be disclosed outside the Department of Veterans Affairs (VA) only if the disclosure is authorized under the Privacy Act, including the routine uses identified in the VA system of records, 58VA21/22, Compensation, Pension, Education and Rehabilitation Records–VA, published in the Federal Register. The requested information is considered relevant and necessary to determine maximum benefits under the law. Information submitted is subject to verification through computer matching programs with other agencies.

RESPONDENT BURDEN: Public reporting burden for this collection of information is estimated to average 15 minutes per response, including the time for reviewing instructions, searching existing data sources, gathering and maintaining the data needed, and completing and reviewing the collection of information. Send comments regarding this burden estimate or any other aspect of this collection of information, including suggestions for reducing this burden, to the Clearance Officer (723), 810 Vermont Ave., NW, Washington, DC 20420; and to the Office of Management and Budget, Paperwork Reduction Project (2900-0057), Washington, DC 20503. PLEASE DO NOT SEND THIS FORM OR APPLICATION FOR BENEFITS TO THESE ADDRESSES.

FIRST NAME - MIDDLE NAME - LAST NAME OF VETERAN   SOCIAL SECURITY NO   VA FILE NO.
David   F   Raz   XXX-XX-7777   CXX-XXX-889

The following statement is made in connection with a claim for benefits in the case of above-named veteran:

In response to your recent August 2001 letter please be advise the intent of my letter of February 28, 2001 was to file an Informal Claim as authorized under 38 CFR 3.155. I did not make my intent clear at the time because I did not know that I had to specifically state whether my intention was for a Formal or Informal claim.

My request to amend my original claim to include Post Traumatic Disorder remains firm. My letter of February 28, 2001 was to alert you that I would be filing a Formal Claim once I gathered all the records and medical statements from VA hospitals and private physicians. I am still in the process of seeking these records.

Do not start the adjudication process in 60 days as your letter so indicates. My understanding of 38 CFR 3.155 is that as long as I submit all my evidence and a formal claim prior to February 28, 2002, service connection when granted will be effective February 28, 2001.

I CERTIFY THAT the statements on this form are true and correct to the best of my knowledge

SIGNATURE David Raz
DATE SIGNED September 3, 2001
ADDRESS 909 Spruce Drive, Tampa, Florida 34703
TELEPHONE NUMBERS 727-555-1212

PENALTY The law provides severe penalties which include fine or imprisonment or both, for the willful submission of any statement or evidence of a material fact, knowing it to be false.

VA FORM EXISTING STOCKS OF VA FORM 214138
JUN 2000   21-4138 APR 994, WILL BE USED

SEPTEMBER 13, 2001: VETERAN PROVIDES
STATEMENT OF COMBAT DUTY

Figure 3.5 contains David Raz's statement giving a day-by-day account of his duty while in Vietnam. This sworn statement by Sgt. David Raz is in response to the August 24, 2001, letter in which the VA requested a detailed account of his combat experiences.

The more facts you can remember and present in an orderly sequence, the better your chances are of having your claim approved. You probably have many memories that you would prefer not to remember because they are too painful. However painful, you must find a way to make these experiences known.

To ensure that David Raz's statement was given the proper weight, it was submitted as a sworn declaration. A sworn statement submitted to the VA has to be given the same weight as any other form of evidence and cannot be considered hearsay evidence or a nonbinding lay statement. An important note to remember: you can collaborate your military combat experiences by obtaining an after action report for the days of events that caused your PTSD. This information is available under the Freedom of Information Act. Have your congressional representative or senator request the information from the military service involved. It's fifty times faster than if you do it on your own.

Fig. 3.5

Declaration of David Raz

Now comes David Raz being duly sworn states as follows:

1. Social Security Number is XXX-XX-7777 VA Claim No. C-XX-XXX-889

2. The following is an accurate account of the events that I experienced during my combat tour of duty in the Republic of Vietnam.

I arrived in Vietnam **February 14, 1970**. All new replacement troops were given one week training prior to being assigned to a combat unit. I became good friends with Sgt. Potholder; we met while walking to classes on booby traps.

I was assigned to 25th Division 2/22 Mechanized, Company B. I flew out to the Company, which was already out in the field. Sgt. Harvey Camp took me to the company commander. I was assigned to the Platoon in which Sgt. Tango was a squad leader. Sgt. Tango briefed me on daily operations.

March 1, 1970, was my first day in the field. The platoon was searching a brushy area. Suddenly someone yelled that he saw a spider hole cover move. I ran over to it aiming my M-16 at the cover. After tying a rope to the lid we stepped back and pulled the lid off. We yelled "Sin Loi" (give up) and "La Dea" (come here). Slowly a hand came up holding a white handkerchief. A pale but healthy NVA soldier climbed out. He was dressed in black pajamas and he was about 5' 10" tall. He had been hiding in the dark damp hole for three months.

We continued searching the brushy area. There was a loud bang and puff of black smoke came from the bushes in front of my Armored Personnel Carrier (APC). PFC Penny staggered out covered from head to toe with bits of glass and scrap metal. He was put on the Medivac helicopter to the hospital in Cu Chi. That night I did guard duty from 3 AM to 6 AM at our night position.

March 2, the second night in the field I went on an ambush patrol with Sgt. Tango's squad. I lay awake all night scared. However, there was no activity in front of us.

March 3 we were searching an area we knew was booby-trapped. The enemy ties grass in three tuffs or places three stones in a triangle as a warning for the local people to avoid the area. We understood these signs but had to go in and search in spite of the possibility of booby traps. In this area I was guarding a tunnel entrance at the bottom of a bomb crater. A grenade rolled up beside me with the pin pulled. I yelled "Oh shit!" The grenade was old and didn't explode.

Later I saw a pile of fresh human excrement. I yelled "gook out of hole". Then a young man in black shorts took off running. The soldiers in front of me shot him dead. We continued our search. Suddenly there was a large explosion over a little hill in front of me. "Damn, who got it now" I said as I rushed over the hill. On the ground lay Lt. Deer and PFC Ruth, the radioman. Lt. Deer was dead as his legs were shredded and his forehead hinged open. His whole brain was lying on the ground. It looked like PFC Ruth was just knocked out because no blood was visible. The medic did mouth-to-mouth and I did CPR on PFC Ruth. As I pushed on his chest his throat gurgled and his blood oozed out onto my hands from a thin cut about 2" long. Shrapnel had hit him in the middle of his sternum - dead. Shaken I had to carry on and prepare Lt. Deer's body for transport. I closed his forehead flap and eyes. I searched his clothes for personal effects. His wallet was full of blood and inside was a picture of his beautiful blond wife and his two young daughters along with $620. I ask someone why he had so much money. He was to leave the next day on R&R in Hawaii to meet his wife and daughters. Next, I dug a hole and buried Lt. Deer's brain. I wanted to fall down and cry but couldn't let my men see my weakness. I took over as Platoon Leader until another Lieutenant could be assigned.

March 17 I went on an ambush patrol outside of Cu Chi with the squads of Sgt. Potholder and Sgt. Villa. After setting up we were attacked by RPGs and AK-47 fire. Hearing the RPGs launched and waiting for them to land was horrifying. Sgt. Potholder had been outside the crater setting up a claymore mine when he was killed.

April 15 we headed up to Tay Ninh near the Cambodian border.

May 4 we finally crossed into Cambodia. We had five fire fights that day.

May 6 we were the lead APC advancing along the edge of the jungle. As we came to a bend in the road the Company Commander told us to hold up. The APCs behind us were having trouble getting through a river. Not being able to see around the bend bothered me. I sent PFC Vic to look around the bend in the trail. He came running back saying the NVA were setting up a large ambush for us. I ordered everyone to fire low, straight ahead and to the right into the jungle. After a couple of minutes we stopped. I asked the Platoon Leader if we could search the jungle. He said no since we had to meet up with another Company before dark. A week later we came past this same spot. The stench was terrible. I guessed we killed a few of them.

May 8 we were traveling through an open field when the Company Commander ordered us to turn right and get on line. We dismounted and walked behind the APCs. Suddenly 2 RPGs exploded in front of the APC next to me. Everyone returned fire. There was so much noise you couldn't tell when they stopped shooting at us. Eventually we came to a long trench 5 feet deep leading into the jungle. It was another hit & run ambush. No one was hurt but there were plenty of bullet marks on our APCs.

May 10 is Mother's Day. My family is giving presents to Mom and settling down to a nice dinner. I am getting ammo and equipment together for a night ambush.

May 24 my brother Paul graduates from High School. The whole family, parents, my other brother, two sisters, aunts, uncles and cousins would all be together. Again, I prepare for a night ambush.

May 30 is Memorial Day. From now on this day is especially personal.

May 31 begins Operation "Bramble Bush." It is a battalion size assault on a large jungle covered hill. As we turned off the road and headed into the jungle, the APC in front of me hit a mine. Two men were injured and Medivaced to the hospital. We continued busting through the jungle. The lead APC in Company C was hit by three RPGs. The driver was severely wounded and the 50 cal. gunner on top of the APC was hit and fell inside. The APC burned with ammo exploding everywhere. The mission continued after a short delay to Medivac the driver to the hospital. All that was left of the gunner could fit in a small bag. Later I was walking behind my APC. I heard noise behind me, I dropped down, took aim with M-16 on auto. As I started to squeeze the trigger I recognized the Captain of Company B leading a squad through the jungle up to the front. I almost killed some of my own men.

At the front, PFC Penny (already wounded by booby trap on March 1st) had been hit. The full front of his skull and face were blown away.

June 2 Sgt. Tango and PFC Rash who I considered my best friends in Vietnam came by to visit. Sgt. Tango asked if I had any clean clothes. Their clothes were totally rotten. I only had 2 shirts, which I gave them. Rash gave me Gouda cheese in a red round wrapper he had received in a package from home that day.

That night Sgt. Stone and I took out an ambush, as did Sgt. Tango. After dark I heard a short burst of AK-47 fire and loud boom from the area where Sgt. Tango took his squad. Someone said "Boy, that was a short fight." PFC Rash had taken many AK-47 bullets in his chest. He was dead before he hit the ground. An RPG hit Sgt. Tango and blew a big hole in his right side. He fell behind a large log and bled to death before they found him. My two best friends were dead in one instant. I cried and threw Rash's Gouda cheese into the jungle. I couldn't eat that cheese now.

June 3 in the middle of the night our night camp was mortared twice. Two soldiers needed to be Medivaced to the hospital with wounds.

June 13 my company was one of the last to leave Cambodia. I was exhausted, dirty, sad and in a daze.

June 15 we had a ceremony to honor all the soldiers who died in Cambodia. Metals were also awarded. I received the Army Commendation medal for meritorious achievement against the enemy.

June 18 I moved to Fire Support base Buel. We escorted a supply convoy every day. It was an easier job and we badly needed the break.

July 1 I went to French Fort Barbara. I took out ambush patrols every night.

July 9 I moved to Katum, which was a mud hole. It was a heavy artillery fire support base that pounded the enemy all night long. At night I lay on my poncho and propped my head up out of the muck.

July 21 two of our Company's APCs hit mines. No one was injured but the tracks on the APCs were damaged.

July 22 I received a letter on a brown paper towel from Sgt. Ronald, a friend from NCO school. He wrote that he has been wounded twice and our friends Sgt. Lester - KIA, Sgt. Mats - KIA, Sgt. Donald - WIA, and Sgt. Bee - WIA. Damn war kept killing my friends.

August 1 I moved back to Cu Chi area. Battalion Commander wasn't getting enough "kills" in his contest with other Commanders. He came up with a plan for Sgt. Camp, Sgt. Falcon and I to be dropped by helicopter deep in the jungle near enemy camps after which we were to "wander around" for three days as targets to draw an attack by NVA troops. Then the Commander could send in Cobra gunships to kill "Gooks" and raise his tally. He didn't care what happened to us. We did a good job of hiding.

August 15 my girlfriend back home married someone else. It was a "Dear John" all the way.

August 18 I was hospitalized. I had lost 30 lbs. and was too weak to function. I also had a parasitic infection - Giardiasis. After many tests, some good food and rest I was sent back to the field on September 4.

September 6 my squad was searching a tall grassy area. An explosion pounded me with shrapnel everywhere. I felt great pain on my face and left eye. I covered my eyes with both hands for fear I was blind. After what felt like an eternity, I moved my hands and was relieved that I could see but there were pieces of metal lodged in my left eye and left temple.

Lying down next to me was Sgt. Stone moaning in pain. His right eye was slowly oozing down his cheek with a massive amount of blood. I put a wad of gauze over the hole where his eye used to be and wrapped his head tightly with gauze. PFC Wider had a piece of shrapnel in his right buttock. We were all Medivaced to the 12th EVAC hospital in Chu Chi. I had my Purple Heart but luckily without losing my sight.

September 9 I was back in the field.

September 14 my APC hit a mine. I was thrown up into the air and fell back down on to the APC. I was bruised and dazed but scrambled for my M-16 thinking we were under attack. We were not under attack; it was just a mine planted alongside a trail. The APC driver injured his eardrums and the APC was damaged.

September 17–24 I went to Taipei, Taiwan for R&R. I was so nervous all the time because I was alone and did not have my M-16. However, I was thankful the food was terrific and I slept in a real bed.

September 27 I was reassigned to do security on top of Nui Ba Den (Black Virgin) mountain. The base was a major communication link for our troops. Another function of this base was for radio and translation personnel to eavesdrop on NVA transmissions. I was in charge of a bunker on the perimeter on top of the mountain. Two PFCs and I had guard duty 24 hours a day in the bunker. At night we fired our M-16 in the semi-automatic position three times every 30 minutes down the edge of the mountain in front of our bunker. If we fired in the automatic position it was a signal that we were under attack.

October 29 Typhoon Louise hit us. It was impossible to see in front of our bunker because of the wind and heavy rain. We all were very nervous that entire night.

November 12 the security of Nui Ba Den Mountain was turned over to the South Vietnamese Army. (ARVN) I was awarded the Army Commendation Award with Oak Leaf Cluster for making improvements in my bunker and providing solid security in my sector.

November 18 I was reassigned to the 1st Cavalry Division. The 25th Division went home to Hawaii. I ended up in Company A of 2/7 Cavalry. Now I was a foot soldier carrying a heavy backpack with ammo and supplies. I had to learn quickly the new operating procedures with a new squad. I became squad leader in a different kind of war.

December 5 I was informed I received a "school drop" of 55 days so I could enroll in college for the spring semester.

December 13 I received a Bronze Star for outstanding meritorious service against hostile forces from February to December 1970.

December 17, 1970, I flew out of Vietnam to Oakland Air Force Base in California. After 22 hours of continuous tests and paperwork, I received my Honorable Discharge.

3. Under penalties of law, I declare that all statements made in this account of my Vietnam experiences are true.

Signature of David Raz   Date

STATE OF FLORIDA COUNTY OF PINELLAS

Sworn to (or affirmed) before me this _____ day of _____, by and in the presence of these witnesses: Witness:
Witness:
Sign Print Personally Know.; OR Produced Identification Type of Identification Produced

OCTOBER 19, 2001: DR. JONES SENDS RESPONSE TO VA[3]

Dr. Jones sent the VA a very detailed account (see figure 3.6) of the severity of David Raz's PTSD. He pointed out that to give Mr. Raz even partial relief from the effects of chronic and permanent PTSD, he would have to remain on Zoloft and Ativan for life. Dr. Jones states David's condition is directly related to his wartime service and meets the 70% disability VA rating standard. Dr. Jones's letter to the VA is an excellent example of the information, style, and depth that is necessary to coax the VA to pay attention to a claim. By law claim processors are required to identify the evidence they have that is superior to a professional physician findings. They cannot simply whip out a phrase like, "a preponderance of evidence is against your claim; therefore, your claim for PTSD is denied." Even though case law mandates how evidence should be weighted, you will see as the chain of events unravels in Sergeant Raz's claim, they actually had denied the claim with this kind of evidence of record.

Fig. 3.6

ADULT AND ADOLESCENT PSYCHIATRY
FORENSIC PSYCHIATRY AND HYPNOTHERAPY

HENRY JONES M.D., PA.
OIL DRUID ROAD EAST- SUITE 3O
CLEARWATER, FL 33756

October 19, 2001

RE: David Raz 5511 XXX—XX—7777

To Whom It May Concern:

    I have been treating Mr. Raz since March 25, 1997. Initially he came to see me because of "job stress". Past history revealed that he had problems with both his mother and his father, who physically abused him as well as the rest of the siblings. He served in the Armed Forces in Vietnam and was actively involved in combat and saw many of his friends killed. This affected him. He was wounded by shrapnel in 1970, his left temple and left eye were injured. His complaints were chest tightness, shallow breathing, upset stomach, loose bowels, as well as depression and anxiety of a long standing nature. He had many posttraumatic symptoms in the Service. He left the Service in 1970, contracted Giardia Lamblia. In 1984 he had a period of weakness for 6 weeks duration, lie exhibited GI malfunction sometime during his life. In 1995, he had his gallbladder removed with some relief of his symptomatology. In 1974 he had a hernia operation. In 1961 he broke his ankle. In 1970, as stated above, he received a shrapnel wound of his left eye and left temple. In 1964, he hit his head while playing basketball and was unconscious for 3 or 4 minutes.

    He never smoked. He drinks about 2 beers a month. His present condition is a build up of life long events, a very bad childhood with parental physical abuse from both parents that continued until he was 16 years of age. He never got along with his parents, although he respected them and feared them. There was no affection between he and his parents and they were very critical of his behavior. His teachers were strict. He had a hard time while he was in the Service and saw active duty in Vietnam.

He married on October 23, 1971, this was his only marriage. He has three children and they are all adults, two girls and one boy. He was honorably discharged from the Service and was a Staff Sergeant and made the rank of E—6. He has never had a pension, although he deserved one. He has worked as a Postal Employee all of his life as a letter carrier. He was interested in art work and cabinetry throughout his life. On March 30, 2001, I wrote a letter to W. Johnson, R.N. of the U.S.P.S. Suncoast District, Occupational Health Services. A copy of this letter is enclosed for your review. At that time I stated that I had been treating Mr. Raz since March 25, 1997 and I felt that he had the following diagnosis:

> 308.3   Acute Posttraumatic Stress Disorder
> 309.81 Chronic Posttraumatic Stress Disorder
> 309.1   Depressive Reaction Prolonged

After a period of not working, at my recommendation, the Post Office felt that he was ready to assume his duties as a Postal Employee. During the time of his not working for the Post Office, he was also treated by Dr. Brown, M.D. of the Orthopedic Associates of West Florida, P.A. He was being treated for a Chronic Disc Disease between C5 and C6 and Degenerative Joint Disease of the SC joint, right shoulder. He was asymptomatic at the time of my writing this letter, as far as his orthopedic problem is concerned. He has to watch himself and may need more treatment in the future, although at the time he began working again he was recovered from that condition, as well as the condition that I have been treating him *for* since 1997.

He has two brothers and two sisters. One brother is 49 years of age and the second brother is 46 years of age. He has a sister who is 54 years of age and another sister who is 50 years of age. David is the oldest sibling. He stated that his parents, as well as his siblings, have had depression. His combat experiences in Vietnam have resulted in Jude's Posttraumatic Stress Disorder. He has had symptoms throughout the years, with symptoms of hyper—vigilance, bad dreams, and other symptoms.

He has been treated by many doctors, but Dr. David Johnson, M.D. has been the one that has been following him and helped him with his parasitic infection, which I think he initially contracted in the Service.

He never graduated from college, although he has some college experiences. I began seeing him in 1997 because he was having trouble at the Post Office.

"According to the "Code of Federal Regulations", revised as of July 1, 2000, Section 38, Part 4, §3.304(f), Mr. Raz does meet the criteria specified. He carries DSM—IV diagnostic codes of 308.3, 309.81 and 309.1, which on page 413 of the above referred manual is listed as code #9411. I feel this is directly related to his experiences while in the Service as described above. His Post—traumatic Stress Disorder is in need of large doses of Ativan and Zoloft from time to time when he experiences PTSD symptoms." Mr. Raz is being treated by me with medication, as well as psychotherapy. I feel that he is 15% disabled.

If you need any further information regarding this individual, please do not hesitate to communicate with me.

Sincerely,

Henry Jones
Henry Jones, M.D.

Part II: 2002

JANUARY 15, 2002: VETERAN RECEIVES THE VA RATING DECISION
After waiting ten months, the VA finally rates David's claim.[4] Figure 3.7 shows the official rating decision issued by the St. Petersburg Regional Office. The January 15, 2002, rating decision denied service connection for PTSD. The reason given for the denial: his service records were silent as to any combat service. It should be noted that the VA rating dated January 9, 1973, granted service connection for David Raz's shell fragment wound—scars upper eyelid and left scalp. He earned a Purple Heart prior to leaving Vietnam. This rating alone should qualify the claim as well grounded, thereby accepting the current claim for PTSD with a lay statement. Development of the claim by the VA should have stopped here. The veteran's lay statement would have been sufficient to move the process along.

1/15/02	Fig. 3.7

NAME OF VETERAN	SOCIAL SECURITY NR
David Raz	XXX-XX 7777

ISSUE:

Service connection for POST TRAUMATIC STRESS DISORDER (PTSD).

EVIDENCE:

Service medical records from 01-23-69 to 12-19-70

DECISION:

Service connection for Post Traumatic Stress Disorder is **denied**.

REASONS AND BASES:

There is no record of POST TRAUMATIC STRESS DISORDER (PTSD) showing a chronic disability subject to service connection. In order to establish service connection, it is necessary to provide evidence which demonstrates the existence of the claimed condition and its possible relationship to service.

The service medical records for the period 01-23-69, through 12-19-70, were carefully reviewed. There is no evidence of any type of psychiatric disability or problem. There is no evidence of any indication of treatment for any disabilities such as anxiety or insomnia; the records are entirely silent for any nervous problems.

The discharge papers show the veteran received a Bronze Star Medal.*

The veteran was sent a letter dated 08-24-01, for additional information before process his claim for PTSD. As of this date, he has not responded to the questions asked in that letter. He was sent another letter of the same date advising him what evidence would be necessary to evaluate his claim. The veteran was advised he had 60 days in which to respond. The veteran did respond stating he filed an informal claim and was not prepared to submit additional evidence at this time. He stated he believed he had until one year from the date of the original claim to submit evidence. The veteran may submit evidence at any time. However, if he would like to protect his date of claim, 03-01-01 (date of receipt of claim), he must respond to the letters of 08-24-01, no later than 08-24-02.

Service connection for PTSD is denied as there is no evidence of a stressor or evidence showing the veteran has this condition.

The rule regarding benefit of reasonable doubt does not apply because the preponderance of evidence is unfavorable.

---

*   Department of Defense Code of Federal Regulation (32 *CFR* Subchapter F, Part 578 §578.11) states: "The Bronze Star is awarded to any individual who has distinguished himself or herself by heroic or meritorious achievement in connection with military operations against armed enemy. For heroism a Valor Device is added to award. For meritorious operation against armed enemy there is no 'V' device requirement." However, according to the VA, to concede a combat stressor the veteran's Bronze Star must also have a "V" device. This policy was put into effect when VA manual M 21 Part VI was changed on October 28, 1998. The VA has been slammed by the U.S. Court of Appeals for Veterans Claims and the U.S. Court of Appeals for the Federal Circuit for establishing a standard that exceed the statutory limits imposed by Congress.

Let's examine a few inaccuracies in this rating decision. Yes, they did send David two letters dated August 24, 2001. One outlined their responsibility in assisting the veteran in developing his claim. The other was a request for information concerning the events that may have caused the alleged PTSD.

As I pointed out, Sergeant Raz was wounded by shrapnel, which the VA rated as service-connected in 1970. This is where the process should have concluded. However, the veteran responded within twenty days of the letter looking for background facts about his combat experiences. One month after David submitted his response, Dr. Jones sent a detailed evaluation to the VA. Now, according to the rating board, there was no evidence in the file supporting his claim five months later? How can that be?

JANUARY 23, 2002: DR. HENRY JONES SUBMITS SECOND STATEMENT

David requested Dr. Jones prepare an assessment of his progress since the last evaluation was submitted to the VA. The purpose of his letter (see figure 3.8) was to show that David's condition was unchanged since Dr. Jones submitted his first evaluation. Dr. Jones emphasized David's condition was not only chronic but permanent.

ADULT AND ADOLESCENT PSYCHIATRY
FORENSIC PSYCHIATRY AND HYPNOTHERAPY

Fig. 3.8

HENRY JONES M.D., PA.
1234 ROAD EAST DRIVE SUITE 1301
CLEARWATER, FL 37366

As stated previously I have been treating Mr. Raz since March 25, 1997. He came to see me initially because of Job stress. In reviewing significant past history, it is noted that Mr. Raz was wounded in Vietnam by shrapnel in 1970; his left eye and left temple were injured. His complaints at that time were chest tightness, shallow breathing, upset stomach, loose bowels, as well as depression and anxiety of long-standing. He had many of the Post-Traumatic symptoms in the Service. While in the Service he also contracted Giardia Lamblia, He left the Service in 1970.

Past physical: history revealed that he broke his ankle in 1960. In 1974 he had a hernia operation. In 1984 he had periods of weakness for 6 weeks duration. He exhibited gastrointestinal malfunctions during his lifetime. In 1995 he had a gallbladder removed, which relieved some of his symptomatology.

In 1970 he received the shrapnel wound to the left eye and left temple. I feel this was significant in the onset of his Post-Traumatic Stress Disorder, as well as the many experiences he had in the Service. This would include many near death experiences and wading in the jungle, many tines in water up to his shoulders.

During my treatment: of Mr. Raz I have diagnosed him with the following:

308.3 Acute Post-Traumatic Stress Disorder
309.81 Chronic Post-Traumatic Stress Disorder
309.1 Depressive Reaction, Prolonged

According to the Code of Federal Regulation Part 3 3.304(f) and Part 4 §4.131, revised as of July 1, 2000, under Rating Schedule 9411, David's depression in not a separate disability, but is a symptom of his Post-Traumatic Stress Disorder. I consider this individual to have a disability, the percentage of which depends on how active his Post-Traumatic Stress Disorder becomes. More recently when he was unable to work for those two months, I would consider him 100% disabled. However, that changed and he has been able to function at work, however, with great stress to him. He requires both Ativan and Zoloft for his Post-Traumatic Stress Disorder and has been taking these medications for years with some alleviation of his symptomatology. Throughout my treatment of him, there have been times when he reacted to spontaneous noises while he was delivering mail and this precipitates Post-Traumatic Stress Disorder symptomatology.

I considered him as having functioned while he has been working, although with great stress due to the Post-Traumatic Stress Disorder. This disorder has at times made itself felt to the point where he becomes incapacitated. This has occurred at least twice during my treatment of him.

I have been treating Mr. Raz with medications as stated above and psychotherapy sessions on a regular basis for his Post-Traumatic Stress Disorder. I would consider his condition not only *chronic*, but *permanent*.

If you need any further information regarding this patient, please do not hesitate to communicate with me.

Sincerely,

Henry Jones
Henry Jones, M.D.

FEBRUARY 15, 2002: VETERAN'S WIFE SUBMITS
SWORN STATEMENT

David Raz's wife crafted this sworn statement, shown in figure 3.9. To demonstrate the social interaction between the veteran, his family, friends, and acquaintances, his wife agreed to give a declaration of her observations during their thirty-two years of marriage. Before preparing her statement, she was briefed that she should avoid giving any kind of opinions, especially medical. This is an important point to remember when obtaining statements from spouses, family, and friends. For example, they should not say "he has PTSD." That statement is reserved for a medical professional. However, they can say, "He wakes up every night in a cold sweat." This is an observation.

If a family member gives an opinion that, for example, the veteran has PTSD, the rating board will throw out the statement because diagnoses cannot be made by a lay person. However, this outcome can be easily sidestepped by ensuring that her statement simply describes the symptoms she observed. She can say that he has nightmares and keeps her up all night. See chapter 2 for a complete list of symptoms associated with PTSD. Mrs. Raz's declaration is an excellent illustration for a spouse or friend to use.

Fig. 3.9

Declaration of Donna Lea Raz

Now comes Donna Lea Raz being duly sworn states as follows:

My name is Donna Lea Raz; I am the wife of David Raz.

 I met David on March 21, 1971 while attending college in San Antonio, Texas. I was attracted to his exuberance for life and love of adventure. He told me he had recently returned from Vietnam and was studying art at St. Mary's. We were married in San Antonio on October 23, 1971 and moved to Clearwater, Florida in May of 1972.

 When we were dating David became easily frustrated if things didn't go as planned. Several times he had outbursts of rage where he would take a baseball bat and smash sculptures he had made in art class. He rarely spoke about Vietnam except in reference to his bout with intestinal parasites. His delicate stomach restricted what type of food he could eat and it was necessary to always be close to a bathroom. In April of 1971, before we were married David visited the VA hospital in San Antonio about his intestinal problem. They said that there was nothing wrong and that it was just stress from being in Vietnam and in time it would get better.

 After we were married his outbursts of anger became more frequent. He had recurring nightmares about Vietnam and would need to check the outside of the house frequently during the night. He was uncomfortable sleeping without a weapon in his hands but he was afraid to have any gun in our house because he didn't trust his learned instinct to kill. He put a large machete under the bed—just in case. As time passed David began to talk a little more about Vietnam but not with specifics. In general he was upset that he had to participate in a war that was like no other in American history. He often expressed and still does that he should not have come home alive. Too many of his buddies died unnecessarily and he felt that he should have gone with them. He felt guilty that he lived and they didn't. No one could understand just how horrible it was to have had that experience. It seemed like he could never stop thinking about Vietnam but would rarely talk about it. Even after counseling at the VA in St. Petersburg, FL in 1973 his Vietnam experiences always haunted him.

 David's gastrointestinal problems did not get better with time. In July of 1972 he was hospitalized with severe intestinal distress. Dr. Raisin treated him in Morton Plant Hospital in Clearwater, Florida. The diagnosis was severe Gastroenteritis. He was discharged and referred to Dr. Duck, General Practitioner, in Largo, Florida. His symptoms persisted and he finally went to the VA Bay Pines Hospital in St. Petersburg, Florida. He spent several weeks there undergoing tests. They could not find anything physically wrong and referred him to a psychiatrist.

 I don't remember if David met with the psychiatrist alone but we met as a couple with Dr. Dell several times over about three months. We talked in general about David's behavior at home. His mood swings how he would fly off the handle at the smallest thing. He would correct me on every little thing I did – how to hold the spoon while cooking, how to park the car just right etc. He couldn't understand any problem I had. My life was just fine as far as he was concern and I had no right to complain. I don't remember ever discussing Vietnam during these sessions.

 After several meetings the psychiatrist suggested David join group therapy. We met with the group once and then David was to continue on his own. He went once or twice but quit because he had little in common with others in the group. David had a family and was struggling to fit into normal society. Most of the other men in the group were alcohol or drug dependent and many had criminal records. David couldn't relate.

In the fall 1974 David began working for the US Post Office as a mail carrier. His stomach was still very sensitive and this caused problems at work since he needed to use the bathroom frequently. Most of the time he was lucky to have a friendly customer or was on a route that had a public restroom.

David's intestinal problems became a major focus for our family. I had to cook just a certain way or he would get sick. He became emotionally upset whenever his intestinal problems would flare – and that was almost daily. Often he would think someone was trying to poison him or put glass in his food to make him sick. Doctors could never find anything wrong and attributed his intestinal problems to mental stress. This only made his emotional instability worse. I would try to cook bland food as often as possible. Whenever we ate out it was an ordeal on what to order. Rarely did the meal settle well and he would go on a tirade about how they put garbage in restaurant food and we could be poisoned. His moods were erratic. He would get upset about something one day and the same thing wouldn't bother him another. Dr. Dragon's explanation was "he is predictably unpredictable". Finally in 1999 he had his gall bladder removed and the severe gastrointestinal distress was relieved. However, to this day all he really likes to eat is a homemade meal of ground beef patty, some form of potato, frozen corn and applesauce. His emotional problems continued.

Under the care of Psychiatrist Dr. Dragon, David was treated with various drugs for his emotional problems. Several different treatments were tried. Some just made him sleep all the time, others made him easier to live with but David didn't like how the drugs made him feel. He felt like he had lost control of himself and his mind was foggy and not "sharp". He eventually stopped taking the medications and no longer saw Dr. Dragon.

David's medical treatment was very costly and put a financial strain on our family. I worked off and on from the beginning of our marriage and permanently since 1985. It was difficult to raise the children, work and deal with David's physical and mental problems. In August of 1978 at the age of 27 we discover that I had a defective heart valve making me tire quickly. The Mitral Stenosis became worse over the years and on September 7, 1997 I had emergency open-heart surgery to implant an artificial mitral valve. While this procedure saved my life, I must continue to take drugs that make me move slowly and my overall stamina is reduced.

We have three children: a daughter born 3/26/73, a son born 7/24/75 and another daughter born 8/22/78. David tried very hard to be a good father to his children. He didn't want them to know much about his being in the army and killing people in war. He did what he thought a good father should—helped with sport teams, went camping and disciplined them when they didn't do as he told them. His discipline was emotionally harsh. He would yell, scream, slam doors, break things and frighten them. They were frightened enough of his outbursts of anger that they became masters at tiptoeing around him. They knew I did the same and we supported each other as we "walked on eggs" when he was in one of his moods. Whenever one of the children got hurt while playing, David's first reaction was to get angry with them. A scraped knee would get a verbal lashing. They would try to hide their injuries until they could find me. I would take care of it and we would downplay what happened.

Our children were very active in sports, participating in community teams for swimming, diving, baseball, soccer, track and other sports in middle school and high school. At sporting events David was the parent to get kicked out of the stadium for harassing the officials. He would get so emotionally involved with the competition that he became belligerent. The children were embarrassed to have him at their activities.

Our children have always had a difficult time talking to their father and could never confide in him. They would talk to me first and I would have to relay only what we felt was necessary so he would not get upset and go into an angry rage. They are now adults living in different states and they still find it difficult to talk to their father. Telephone conversations are very brief and superficial.

From the days of our early marriage until the present David is easily irritated by small inconveniences of daily life. I can't wait in lines as he becomes very irritated. He can't handle traffic and is prone to road rage. Consequently I do all the driving whenever possible. On January 7, 2001 we moved our daughter's belongings to Atlanta with a U-Haul truck. David was unable to handle the stress and I drove the truck the entire distance.

Any movie or TV show that contains emotional issues or violence can set him off. Images can stay with him for weeks and he will have nightmares. As recently as February of 2001 he was watching a show—Dateline or some other "issue conscious" program. He was total wrapped up in the subject matter. He became visibly upset and enraged about our unfair legal system. His voice was quivering and kept shaking his head. I had to get him to turn off the TV and remind him not to watch this type of show. We limit our viewing to comedies, nature documentaries, and westerns and "light" subject matter.

David has a difficult time socializing. He is very cynical and frequently challenges other's statements on any subject and becomes argumentative. If the topic of war comes up he usually will not join the conversation and walk away. We have only a few friends. During a New Year's Day party we attended together this January, he didn't want to talk with anyone and preferred to sit in the corner watching the football games by himself. He prefers to do solitary work and is excellent at woodworking.

In of March 1997 David had some trouble with his job. I don't know what exactly happened but he became extremely upset that he would loose his job and his life would be ruined. He was in an extremely anxious state and sought help from Psychiatrist Dr. Jones. Dr. Jones immediately put him on medication for anxiety and antidepressants. David has seen Dr. Jones on a regular basis ever since. The medicine that David currently takes has kept his emotions fairly stable.

In February of this year David had a run-in with a supervisor at work. He was feeling very stressed at his job and wanted to see Dr. Jones. David gave his supervisor a 2-week notice for time off to see the doctor but they gave him a hard time about taking this sick leave. There was some exchange of words and David left work immediately to see Dr. Jones. The doctor put him on immediate leave due to stress. David's medications were increased and he visited Dr. Jones weekly. For the first time in a couple of years, David began to talk about Vietnam. This time he was more graphic then ever about what he saw and did there. He also expressed deep feelings of survivor guilt.

Currently, David is back to work at the Post Office and is seeing Dr. Jones every other week.

Signature of Donna Lea Raz
Date

FEBRUARY 19, 2002: VETERAN FILES NOTICE OF DISAGREEMENT

On February 19, 2002, David Raz served a Notice of Disagreement (NOD) to the VA disagreeing with the January 28, 2002, denial of benefits. He used VA Form 21-4138, also used earlier to put the VA on notice about the claim date. He stated the effective date of the award (figure 3.4) was erroneous. He also restated that the VA was advised on September 3, 2001, that an informal claim was filed February 28, 2001. Attached to this NOD were three sworn statements by the veteran (figure 3.10), his wife (figure 3.9), and an addendum from Dr. Jones's medical evaluation (figure 3.8).

Fig. 3.10

Declaration of David Raz*

Now comes David Raz being duly sworn, states as follows:

1.   My name is David Raz. I reside at 909 Spruce Drive, Tampa, FL. 34701

2.   My VA Claim number is C-XX-XXX-889 and SS number is XXX-XX-7777.

3.   I was inducted into the United States Army on March 13, 1969 and served honorably until I was discharged on December 19, 1970. When separated from the Army I was a sergeant grade E-5. I served in the Republic of Vietnam from February 14, 1970 to December 18, 1970. The following medals and awards were earned during my service: Bronze Star, Combat Infantry Badge, Army Commendation Medal with one oak leaf cluster, Purple Heart, National Defense Service Medal, Vietnam Service Medal

4.   On September 6, 1970, I received shrapnel wound to the left upper eyelid and left scalp which are evidenced by scars.

5.   The combat military experiences that were the genesis of my PTSD are addressed in a separate statement.

6.   My post service experiences as they relate to PTSD are detailed in the following paragraphs:

I arrived home in Floral Park, Illinois December 18th, 1970. I was weak, having lost 30 pounds, jumpy, nervous and felt vulnerable without a weapon. It was great to be out of Vietnam but I was constantly nauseated and very uncomfortable. I decided to use my GI Bill and attend college. I moved to San Antonio, Texas to attend College. Every night before going to bed I had to walk around my garage apartment carrying a broom handle for a weapon.

Having checked my perimeter I went to bed clutching the broom handle to my chest like I did my M-16 in Vietnam. I would wake up 10 times a night at the slightest sound. Nightmares of Vietnam bothered me. I would dream that I was in a battle and my M-16 wouldn't fire or that I was chasing "gooks" through a swamp and my legs would get stuck in the marsh and I couldn't get out. I felt miserable.

One day I was riding my motorcycle down a highway at 60 mph when a nearby car backfired. I started to jump off the motorcycle to "get low for fire" but caught myself at the last moment. That incident scared me and from then on I tried to be careful about reacting to loud noises. I went to the VA in San Antonio with symptoms of nausea, bloating, diarrhea, and nervousness. They told me it was *"just battle fatigue and would heal in time."*

On October 23, 1971 I married Donna Lea Billie in San Antonio, Texas and we have lived as man and wife since that date. What an experience it was for her to witness my nighttime rituals and continuous nightmares. I quit college with only one semester left to graduate and moved to Clearwater, FL in May of 1971.

I remember an incident shortly after we moved to Clearwater, FL. that troubled me for years afterwards. We attended a 4th of July celebration and everything was fine until the fireworks went off. I got very agitated and started to cry as I remembered friends who died in Vietnam. From that day on, I avoided all public ceremonies celebrating events that honored our national dead. Even today, 32 years after leaving Vietnam I can not watch TV shows about Vietnam or listen to people talking on TV about wars. It upset me so that I have to change channels.

I started working for the US Post Office as a mail carrier in 1974. The work environment is very stressful with lots of arguing between supervisors and me on how long it will take me to deliver the mail on a specific day. Daily the tension wears on me. I get moody, sometimes lose my temper, and start yelling and even throwing mail across the room. My fellow workers tease me a lot about being a crazy Vietnam Vet and ask me when I am going to go "Postal." My job as a letter carrier provoked my condition. On two occasions I was off work for six-weeks and most recently for seven-weeks because the stress triggered by my job exacerbated my PTSD disorder.

When our children were involved in baseball and soccer I was the parent who made a scene yelling at the referees and umpires. I am very critical of my wife. I notice everything that is out of place or has a new nick on it. Often I would correct her on the slightest mistake or tell her she did not park the car correctly.

I am super alert to everything around me. When I'm walking on the street I'm always conscious of the people around me. Are they following me, or going to rob me? I can't tolerate having anyone close to me in stores or whenever I stand in a line. In a restaurant, I have to sit with my back to a wall or the smallest number of people. I am always nervous and anxious. I feel like something is wrong but I don't know what.

I have trouble with all authority and I react negatively to their ideas or attempts to boss me around. I have no friends with whom I socialize. I do not have golfing friends, bar buddies, nor bicycle riding buddies. I go alone. I only work my job and come home to work on the house or watch TV. I cannot handle traffic. Long waits at lights or slow moving traffic upsets me. I am prone to road rage and yell at people behind the wheel sometimes following them for 10 or 15 minutes. My wife does all the driving when we go anywhere together, dinner, shopping or long distance trips to visit our children.

Currently, I continue to have dreams about Vietnam. My M-16 will not fire or I cannot move through the swamp fast enough. Sometimes I'm lost and I don't know what to do next.

With the help of Dr. Jones, I am struggling to handle the stresses of everyday life. The medications Zoloft and Ativan have helped somewhat. Nevertheless, I am still having great difficulty living peaceably with my job and family. I have been in therapy for more than five years. Even with this, it is necessary for me to take five one-week vacations each year to remove myself from an environment that triggers a PTSD reaction.

7. Under penalties of law, I declare that all statements made in this account of my post Vietnam experiences are true.

Signature of David Raz
Date
STATE OF FLORIDA COUNTY OF PINELLAS

Sworn to (or affirmed) before me this_____day of _____, by and in the presence of these witnesses: Witness:
Witness

Sign Print Personally Know.; OR Produced Identification Type of Identification Produced:

---

*   This response to the VA letter is a legally binding sworn statement. This is a good example to use whenever you are submitting a written statement to the VA. The VA must now treat this statement as positive evidence supporting your case.

JUNE 26, 2002: VA SENDS LETTER REQUESTING
MORE MEDICAL EVIDENCE

The VA sent the letter shown in figure 3.11 to Dr. Jones in June 2002. This letter is meaningless and without merit considering how much medical background information Dr. Jones had already submitted to the VA on behalf of the veteran. This is the type of letter sent to a veteran's physician when the veteran first files a claim.

This letter also provides another example of the VA extending claim-processing time. By sending a letter to the doctor telling him he has sixty days to reply, the VA can safely ignore this claim until that time period has passed. Once this letter goes out, the file is shipped back to the filing room where it will stay until the computer sends out an alert message that the sixty days have expired.

Prior to sending this request, the VA had more than enough medical evidence to make a decision. Only five months earlier, Dr. Jones provided the VA with an updated medical evaluation of David's condition.

Fig. 3.11

DEPARTMENT OF VETERANS AFFAIRS
St. Petersburg Regional Office
P.O. BOX 1431
St. Petersburg, FL 33731

JUN 26, 2002
Dr. Henry Jones   In Reply Refer To: 3 17/TM75/pec
1234 East Road Drive, Suite 1301
Clearwater, FL 33756

Dear Dr. Jones:

The veteran, David Raz, whose Social Security Number is XXX-XX-7776, has applied
for disability benefits showing treatment by you on or about March 1997 to the present.

We are Requesting Medical Evidence
While it is the responsibility of claimants to furnish evidence required in support of their
claim, it has been our consistent practice to assist all veterans and their dependents in
every way possible. In keeping with this practice, we request, on their behalf, evidence in
the possession of others; as in this case, evidence of the veteran having received medical
treatment from you.

The veteran has consented to your giving us information concerning this treatment and
has waived any privilege which readers such information confidential. Collection of the
information requested is authorized by law (38 CFR 3.326).

We Request This Evidence Within 60 Days
As a service to the veteran we would appreciate you furnishing us a report of your
findings and diagnosis, without charge as there are no funds available to pay for this
service. We request this evidence be furnished as soon as possible, preferably within 60
days from the date of this letter.

When No Evidence Is Available
If no medical evidence is of record, a negative response on your letterhead paper would
be greatly appreciated. While you are not required to respond, your cooperation is needed
to make a determination as to the veteran's entitlement to disability benefits. Please be
sure to show the veteran's full name and VA file number on all correspondence or
evidence submitted. A preaddressed envelope, requiring no postage is enclosed for your
convenience along with a copy of this letter for your records.

Do You Have Questions Or Need Assistance

Sincerely yours,

Henry Jones
Henry Jones, M.D.

AUGUST 19, 2002: DR. JONES RESPONDS TO VA REQUEST

In his response to the VA's June 2002 request, Dr. Jones summarized everything he knew of David since he started treating him in 1997. His letter emphasized that David's condition is not only chronic, but also permanent. He also alerted the VA that events surrounding David could totally incapacitate him at any time. Dr. Jones responded within the sixty-day suspense date, forwarding a five-page complete medical history of David Raz. He once again reviewed David's records obtained under the Freedom of Information Act and could add nothing new. Dr. Jones's report is too long to include in its entirety. The closing paragraph summarizes David's albatross:

> David is someone that I would call a "silent sufferer." He does not verbalize how he is feeling to his wife and/or employer and tries to keep everything bottled up until it explodes in an emotional state. He has had many arguments with his supervisors at work. Before [treatment] with me, he even had developed a plan to do harm to the individuals he felt were threatening him, although he did not carry this plan out. He has many sick days banked and was forced to take medical leave of absence last year due to his Post Traumatic Stress Disorder disability. He strives to be reliable and efficient in his duties. And he also tries to be as flexible as possible with the many demands that are put on him at this job. However, even with medication, the stress of these situations that David has a tendency to "bottle up" becomes too much and his Post Traumatic Stress Disorder disability once again exacerbates, leaving him incapacitated. When he is incapacitated, even simple daily living tasks become hard for him to accomplish.

SEPTEMBER 9, 2002: BAY PINES VAMC SCHEDULES
C&P EXAM FOR PTSD

Figure 3.12 is an example of the standard instructions issued by the medical center conducting the C&P examination. The C&P Exam is probably one of the highest alert areas for any veteran claiming benefits. See chapter 7 for details why everything hinges on this examination. This action by the VA came eighteen months after the claim was filed.

Fig. 3.12

DAVID RAZ
909 Spruce Drive
Tampa, FL 34703

Dear Mr. David Raz,

Your examination for either Compensation or Pension has been scheduled at the
Department of Veterans Affairs Medical Center (VAI4C), Bay Pines, Florida on:

MONDAY SEP 16, 2002 2:00 PM BLDG 22-203 C&P Dallis Clinic

The above appointment has been reserved for you. In an effort to complete your
examination as promptly as possible, we request your cooperation in reporting for this
scheduled appointment. Please report at the designated time and do not leave the clinic
until you are advised that all examinations and diagnostics have been completed. If you
do not report for the exam as scheduled without notifying our office, your examination
request may be returned to the VA Regional Office.

PLEASE COMPLETE PAGE ONE OF THE ENCLOSED YELLOW FORM (REPORT OF
MEDICAL EXAMINATION FOR DISABILITY EVALUATION) PAYING PARTICULAR
ATTENTION TO ITEM 17. IF YOU HAVE ANY QUESTIONS PERTAINING TO THIS
FORM, CONTACT YOUR SERVICE OFFICER OR A VETERANS BENEFITS
COUNSELOR. PLEASE BRING YOUR EYEGLASSES, IF WORN, A1~ID A LIST OF YOUR
CURRENT MEDICATIONS.

The purpose of this exam is to evaluate your present claim for Compensation or Pension.
Medical treatment will NOT be provided during this scheduled examination. If you do
not have a Primary Care provider and plan to seek care at Bay Pines VANC, you MUST
contact our Eligibility Office at 727-398-6661, extension 4165; or, outside Pine as
County, 1-888-820-0230

DAWN C. PROTO, Chief
Health Benefits Administration Service

SEPTEMBER 16, 2002: VAMC CONDUCTS C&P EVALUATION

The results of David Raz's C&P Exam can be found in figure 3.13. When scheduled for a C&P evaluation, cautionary measures must be taken to protect your rights. A detail explanation will be found in chapter 7. However, five points must be repeated over and over:

1. Make sure the examiner has read your entire C-file.
2. Keep track of how long you are with the examiner.
3. Ask the examiner about his or her medical background.
4. If a physician's assistant or a nurse practitioner conducts the exam, be extra vigilant in observing what they do and say.
5. Make certain the examiner follows the medical protocol for the condition being evaluated. (A copy of the C&P Exam for PTSD is provided in chapter 7.)

Fig. 3.13

Compensation and Pension Exam Report   page 1

Bay Pines, Florida
·· REPRINT OF FINAL ··

For INITIAL EVALUATION FOR POST-TRAUMATIC STRESS DISORDER (PTSD) Exam

Name: Raz, David

SSN: XXX-XX-7776 (H7776
C-Number XX-XXX-886
DOB: AUG 18,1943

Address: 909 Spruce Drive
Tampa, FL 34703-2307

Res Phone:813-555-1234
Bus Phone: NONE

Entered active service: MAR 13, 1969
Released active service: DEC 19, 1970

Last rating exam date:

Priority of exam: Other

Examining provider: Dallis, ED

Examined on: SEP 16, 2002

Examination results:

HISTORY:

This is a compensation and pension examination for post-traumatic stress disorder (PTSD). The patient was seen 9/16/02. His appointment time was 2:00 pm. His exam reference number is 63056. This evaluation was based on the results of a clinical interview, and review of his C-File. Mr. Raz is a 59 year old married Caucasian male veteran who served in the Army on active duty between 3/69 and 12/70. During his military service he was in Vietnam in 1970, between 2/14 and 12/18.

PSYCHIATRIC HISTORY:

Mr. Raz was first treated at the Vet Center in St. Petersburg in 1973, where he was involved in group therapy for about a year. He quit that program when he found that he couldn't relate to the group members. He sought treatment in the private sector. He saw Dr. Dragon, a Psychiatrist, for about two years in the early 1980's, and started treatment with Henry Jones. a Psychiatrist in the private sector, in Clearwater. He has been under the care of Dr. Jones since 3/25/97. He first sought treatment because of job stress, but it became clear later on that he was also suffering from PTSD related to his combat experiences in Vietnam. He is seen at this point once every three months, and his medications include Ativan and Zoloft.

MEDICAL HISTORY:

Mr. Raz reports that he is in good health, except that he has high cholesterol, and for that he takes Zocor.

OCCUPATIONAL HISTORY:

Mr. Raz is a letter carrier. He has worked for the Post Office for 27 years, and has been at his current station in Tampa for 13 years. Since he started his medication he has been doing fairly well. The station manager is a very aggressive pusher, and he has some confrontations with her, but he gets along very well with his immediate supervisor who is understanding, and leaves him alone. However, prior to his taking medication he was involved in what he described as bad judgments, and having gotten in arguments, after which they could have fired him. He stated that once when he was upset he threw a tray of mail across the room, and he also verbally attacked his supervisor.

SOCIAL HISTORY:

Mr. Raz has been married since 1971. He and his wife have three adult children (ages 29, 26, and 24). His wife works as a law librarian in the private sector. He states that he is happily married, but his *wife* has health problems which leave her weak, and they have been arguing more lately. They have resided in their current home for 31 years, and are supported by their salaries, and small interest income from their CDs. Financially they are doing just fine, and after having put three children through college, and having sold all their assets to do that, they are now trying to save money for the future. In his leisure time Mr. Raz enjoys working around the house, painting, and doing repairs. Lately he has come home from work, and had to relax because of the heat of the summer. He will watch TV, and go to bed early, but he does enjoy being more active, and also is responsible for cleaning up the yard. Socially, he and his wife go out to eat, and they go shopping. They have made acquaintances through their children's school, and sports activities, but they don't get together socially with any of those people. His wife has girl friends; he himself does not have any friends. They and their children do visit back and forth. He is a member of the Catholic Church, and goes to church on Sundays. He used to be involved in more activities in the past, but during the 1980's he withdrew because he found that he couldn't function in social settings properly.

SUBSTANCES:

Mr. Raz denied any problems with alcohol. He stated that he drank some when he was younger, but he always experienced such a bad hangover that it was never enjoyable for him. He will have an occasional beer. He denied any use of drugs, or tobacco products.

LEGAL HISTORY:

Mr. Raz denied any history of arrests.

MENTAL STATUS EXAMINATION:

Mr. Raz arrived early for his appointment. He is of average height, and was casually dressed in short sleeve cotton knit shirt and shorts. He has short hair, and has a gray beard, and mustache. He was wearing glasses, and he was noted to be wringing his hands throughout much of the session. He presented as a very soft spoken, mild, and mellow individual who established and maintained good eye contact throughout the session. He admitted to some situational anxiety. Cognitively he appeared to be intact. No abnormalities of speech or thought were noted. He denied visual and auditory hallucinations. He admitted to suicidal ideation with possible plan, but without intent because of religious beliefs, and concern for his family. He denied any history of suicide attempts. He admitted to a history of homicidal ideation with a plan, but without intent, again for the same reasons that he would not commit suicide. He has a history of violent behavior, but not toward individuals, rather, in frustration he will break windows or furniture etceteras. This was his behavior before he was stabilized on medication. Insight into his problems is good. Social judgment is good.

MILITARY HISTORY:

Mr. Raz served in the Army, and was involved in combat. When questioned about his worst memories of his experiences in Vietnam he reiterated the events which he already talked about in the report that he wrote which is in the file, so they will not be repeated here.

SUBJECTIVE COMPLAINTS:

Mr. Raz reported problems with a nervous stomach and headaches. He cites problems consistent with hyper vigilance. He watches all people and fears someone will attack him. Small things set off an overreaction and anger during which he may scream, curse, or break things. He avoids social events, and does not talk to people at work. He has no friends. Loud noises startle him, and his heart pounds in his chest, and makes him nervous and anxious at work. During times of stress at work he will take extra medication. He avoids all war movies, and if something comes on the TV having to do with that subject matter, he will change the channel. He is moody and talks very little. Sounds outside of the bedroom window wake him up many times during the night. He has nightmares of being stuck in the jungle, or his M-16 will not fire, or arguing with officers about maneuvers. He is comfortable in a restaurant only if his back is to a wall. He cannot stand to have people stand behind him or walk behind him. He has considered numerous times murder and/or suicide. His wife also wrote a letter of support listing his symptomatology. She stated that he has had outbursts of rage, destroying objects, and is prone to road rage. He has avoided speaking about Vietnam until very recently. Mr. Raz stated that was because people treat Vietnam veterans with less disdain then before. Before, they were known as baby killers and evoked no sympathy. She stated that he slept with a large machete under his bed. He experiences and expresses survivor guilt, he has had flashbacks triggered by smells, or such as something cooking, or years ago when they went on family vacation camping trips, it would remind him of setting up camp in Vietnam. When his children brought home Cambodian friends his first reaction was wanting to shoot them. Helicopters also remind him of his combat experiences. He is irritable and cannot wait in lines. When his children were young, he was kicked out of the stadium of their sporting events for harassing officials. Interpersonally, his wife finds him to be cynical, to be challenging others, argumentative, and if anyone discusses war, he walks away and isolates himself. He prefers solitary work.

DIAGNOSTIC IMPRESSION:

AXIS I: Post-traumatic stress disorder (PTSD)
AXIS II: No diagnosis.
AXIS III: None affecting his psychological functioning; he did have a long term parasitic
          disorder which apparently is cured.
AXIS IV: Exposure to combat, stressful working conditions.
AXIS V: Global Assessment of Functioning (GAF) equals 50. This Global Assessment
of Functioning (GAF) reflects serious symptoms of Post-traumatic stress disorder (PTSD) which affect his psychological well being and social functioning. He is able to manage occupationally through the use of medication and an understanding supervisor. He is competent to manage his own financial affairs.

DD 9-16-02 DT 9-17-02 JOB 200948 TRANS 805/VARO

SEPTEMBER 24, 2002: VA ACKNOWLEDGES RECEIPT OF NOD

The VA claim processors stated that they received the veteran's Notice of Disagreement with their decision of February 19, 2002, and they were proceeding with the appeal process. However, it seems clear that they already had made their minds up to continue the denial of PTSD benefits when the C&P Exam was ordered.

This acknowledgment is dated September 24, 2002, and the date the C&P Exam was completed and forwarded to the RO was September 16, 2002. The results of the C&P Exam failed to convince members on team 70 that the veteran had a legitimate claim for PTSD benefits. The only explanation I can see for this blatant disregard for the results of the C&P Exam is that they had no intention of deciding if David's PTSD disability was related to his service. Instead, team 70 was not going to grant a benefit for PTSD but rather forward the claim to the next level for someone else to make the decision.

Part III: 2003

APRIL 30, 2003: VA GRANTS SERVICE CONNECTION FOR PTSD

The VA advised David that service connection for PTSD was approved, effective April 30, 2003, and his PTSD was rated 70% disabling. However, as shown in the May 20, 2003, award letter in figure 3.14, the rating board considered only evidence dated between January 23, 2002, and September 16, 2002, without explaining why records between February 28, 2001, and October 19, 2001, were not considered relevant to support an entitlement date of March 1, 2001.

You should be alert to a "snake in the grass" when the last paragraph reads like this: "This constitutes a complete grant of benefits sought and this issue is being removed from appeal without further appellate review." With this statement the VA adjudicators were effectively trying to coerce the vet into accepting their decision. If they failed to address all the issues of the claim, as they did in this case, appeal the decision. They can't take away what they granted and they can't stop you from appealing any issues they failed to address. As you will see later, by challenging the rating after they granted a 70% entitlement rate, the veteran ultimately received another $13,000 as back benefits. This is because rating board members overlooked evidence that was in the file from February 28, 2001, to February 28, 2002.

Fig. 3.14

MAY 20 2003

DEPARTMENT OF VETERANS AFFAIRS
St. Petersburg Regional Office
P.O. BOX 1431
St. Petersburg, FL 33731

DAVID RAZ   In Reply Refer To: 317, Post Team I/RJR
909 Spruce Drive   C XX-XXX-887
Tampa, FL 34703   RAZ, D

Dear Mr. Raz:

We made a decision on your Notice of Disagreement received on February 19, 2002.

This letter tells you about your entitlement amount and payment start date and what we decided. It includes a copy of our rating decision that gives the evidence used and reasons for our decision. We have also included information about additional benefits, what to do if you disagree with our decision, and who to contact if you have questions or need assistance.

What Is Your Entitlement Amount And Payment Start Date?

Your monthly entitlement amount is shown below:

Monthly Entitlement Amount	Payment Start	Reason For Change Date
S995.Q0	Feb. 1,2002	initial date of entitlement
1,008.00	Dec 1,2002	cost of living allowance adjustment

We are paying you as a single veteran with no dependents.

When Can You Expect Payment?

Your payment begins the first day of the month following your effective date. You will receive a payment covering the initial amount due under this award, minus any withholdings, in approximately 15 days. Payment will then be made at the beginning of each month for the prior month. For example, benefits due for May are paid on or about June 1.

Rating Decision NAME OF VETERAN	I *Department of Veterans Affairs* St *Petersburg Regional Office*	Page 1 4/30/03
Raz, David		

R VA File Number	SOCIAL SECURIT NR	POA
C XX-XXX-887	XXX-XX-7776	American Legion

INTRODUCTION:

You are a Vietnam Era veteran and served in the U.S Army from 03-13-69, to 12-19-70. We received your Notice of Disagreement on 02-19-02. We grant service connection for a disease or disability that began in service or was caused by some event or experience in service. Based on a review of the evidence listed below, we have made the following decision(s) on your claim.

ISSUE:

Service connection for post-traumatic stress disorder.

EVIDENCE:

Service medical records for the period 01-23-69, through 12-19-70
201 Personnel File from the United States Army
Statements from Dr. Henry Jones dated 01-23-02, and 08-19-02
Two statements from the veteran dated 02-14-02
Statement from the veteran's wife, Donna Lea Raz, dated 02-15-02
Notice of Disagreement received 02-20-02
VA examination dated 09-16-02, from VANC, Bay Pines, FL.

DECISION:

Service connection for post-traumatic stress disorder is granted with an evaluation of 70 percent effective January 23, 2002.

REASONS FOR DECISION:

Service connection for post-traumatic stress disorder has been established as directly related to military service.

A review of your VA claims file shows that rating decision of Ql-l5-O~, denied entitle-ment to service connection for post-traumatic stress disorder as there was no evidence of record of a stressor or medical evidence of a diagnosis of post-traumatic stress disorder.

Since that action was taken, your 201 Personnel File from the United States Army was received. A review of that file shows that you were awarded the Purple Heart, which serves to verify an in-service stressor occurred. Also, you have submitted medical evidence which contains a diagnosis of post-traumatic stress disorder, which the examiner relates to your military service. Therefore, entitlement to service connection for post-traumatic stress disorder is granted.

Statements from Dr. Jones dated 01-23-02, and 08-19-02, provide a lengthy discussion of your personal and medical history. He states that you suffer headaches, hyper alertness and agitation and that you take Ativan and Zoloft four times per day each. He states these medications lessen the severity of your symptoms and that you must take them to control your symptoms. He states that you react to spontaneous noises while you are delivering mail and this precipitates post-traumatic stress disorder symptomatology. He describes you as having functioned while you have been working, although with great stress due to your post-traumatic stress disorder. This disorder has a times made itself felt to the point where you become incapacitated, which he states has occurred at east twice during his treatment of you. Dr. Jones describes times that you have exacerbations that incapacitate you. During these times, he notes that simple daily living tasks at home become hard for you to accomplish. He states that you have missed a great deal of work due to these incapacitating episodes.

Your statements provide extensive detail of your experiences in Vietnam and subsequent to your return from Vietnam. You indicate you were and continue to be anxious, suffer from nightmares. "check the perimeter" before going to bed, and have survivor guilt.

Statement from your spouse describes your relationship with her and your children. She also describes your behavior during social activities, checking your surroundings numerous times nightly, mood swings, job stress, etc.

VA examination shows you see Dr. Jones every three months and are taking Ativan and Zoloft for your post-traumatic stress disorder. Upon examination examiner noted you to wring your hands throughout much of the session. You were very soft spoken, mild and mellow and established good eye contact. You admitted to some situational anxiety. You denied visual and auditory hallucinations. You admitted to suicidal ideation with possible plan. Without intent because of religious beliefs and concern for your family. You denied history of suicide attempts. You admitted to a history of homicidal ideation with a plan, but without intent, again for the same reasons that you would not commit suicide. You spoke of a history of violent behavior, which examiner noted was prior to stabilization on medication. Insight and social judgment were good. A Global Assessment of Functioning (GAF) score of 50 was assigned. Due to the symptomatology of suicidal ideation, incapacitating episodes, ritual of checking the perimeter, anxiety, etc., a 70 percent evaluation is assigned. It is determined that this percentage most accurately reflects your symptomatology.

The effective date is January 23, 2002, the date of medical evidence which first shows a diagnosis of post-traumatic stress disorder. It is noted that you filed your claim much earlier than this date; however, there is **no** medical evidence of a diagnosis of post-traumatic stress disorder before January 23, 2002, in the records available for review.

A higher evaluation of 100 percent is not warranted unless there is total occupational and social impairment due to such symptoms as: gross impairment in thought processes or communication; persistent delusions or hallucinations; grossly inappropriate behavior; persistent danger of hurting self or others; intermittent inability to perform activities of daily living (including maintenance of minima! personal hygiene); disorientation to time or place; memory loss for names of close relatives, own occupation, or own name. Since there is a likelihood of improvement the assigned evaluation is not considered permanent and is subject to a future review examination.

This constitutes a complete grant of benefits sought and this issue is being removed from appeal without further appellate review.

MAY 31, 2003: VETERAN FILES NOTICE OF DISAGREEMENT

The effective date of February 1, 2002, was not the appropriate start date for benefits according to the VA's own regulations. We knew the file contained medical evidence going all the way back to February 28, 2001, when David originally filed his claim for PTSD service connection. Our best guess at why this evidence was ignored is that the rater only reviewed information in the file as far back as January 15, 2002. This was the date the VA denied the original claim for PTSD benefits. This practice is known as "top sheeting." The VA justifies top sheeting because of regulations governing the appeal process. When a claim is denied, the claimant has one year from the date of notification to file an appeal. Once the year has passed, the issued is dead. In our case, the action was improper because the VA adjudicator initially gave us one year from the date of the informal claim, January 28, 2001, to obtain all the evidence and file the original claim. The rater overlooked this fact.

When filing a NOD, it's important that you focus your rebuttal on the issues the VA failed to address and, when you can, cite references to support your rebuttal. To help organize your appeal and keep the facts in focus, it is suggested that you fashion your appeal from the one we filed with the VA on May 31, 2003, which can be seen in figure 3.15. Italics have been added for emphasis.

OMB Approved No. 2900-0075 Respondent Burden: 15 minutes

Fig. 3.15

Department of Veterans Affairs   STATEMENT IN SUPPORT OF CLAIM

PRIVACY ACT INFORMATION: The law authorizes us to request the information we are asking you to provide on this form (38 U.S.C. 501(a)) and (b)). The responses you submit are considered confidential (38 U.S.C. 5701). They may be disclosed outside the Department of Veterans Affairs (VA) only if the disclosure is authorized under the Privacy Act, including the routine uses identified in the VA system of records, 58VA21/22, Compensation, Pension, Education and Rehabilitation Records–VA, published in the Federal Register. The requested information is considered relevant and necessary to determine maximum benefits under the law. Information submitted is subject to verification through computer matching programs with other agencies.

RESPONDENT BURDEN: Public reporting burden for this collection of information is estimated to average 15 minutes per response, including the time for reviewing instructions, searching existing data sources, gathering and maintaining the data needed, and completing and reviewing the collection of information. Send comments regarding this burden estimate or any other aspect of this collection of information, including suggestions for reducing this burden, to the Clearance Officer (723), 810 Vermont Ave., NW, Washington, DC 20420; and to the Office of Management and Budget, Paperwork Reduction Project (2900-0057), Washington, DC 20503. PLEASE DO NOT SEND THIS FORM OR APPLICATION FOR BENEFITS TO THESE ADDRESSES.

FIRST NAME - MIDDLE NAME - LAST NAME OF VETERAN	SOCIAL SECURITY NO	VA FILE NO.
David F Raz	XXX-XX-7777	CXX-XXX-889

The following statement is made in connection with a claim for benefits in the case of above-named veteran:

This Notice of Disagreement is in response to your rating of April 30, 2003. These are the specific issues I disagree with:

Issue 1. No medical evidence to support claim

Statement: "A review of your VA claim file shows that rating of 01—15-02, denied entitlement to service connection for Post Traumatic Stress Disorder as there was no evidence of a stressor or medical evidence of a diagnosis of PTSD."

Rebuttal 1: VA Rating Decision of 06—26-71 grants 0% for Shell Fragment Scars Right Upper Eyelid and Left Scalp. This acknowledgement by VA of a combat injury meets the intent of 38 CFR §3.304(f).

I CERTIFY THAT the statements on this form are true and correct to best of my knowledge

SIGNATURE David Raz

DATE SIGNED May 31, 2003

ADDRESS 909 Spruce Drive, Tampa, Florida 34703

TELEPHONE NUMBERS 727-555-1212   None

PENALTY The law provides severe penalties which include fine or imprisonment or both, for the willful submission of any statement or evidence of a material fact, knowing it to be false.

VA FORM	EXISTING STOCKS OF VA FORM 214138
JUN 2000	21-4138 APR 994, WILL BE USED

Rebuttal 2: The regulation states in part — *"Post Traumatic Stress Disorder:* If the evidence establishes that the veteran engaged in combat with the enemy and the claimed stressor is related to that combat, in the absence of clear and convincing evidence to the contrary, and provided that the claimed stressor is consistent with the circumstances,

conditions, or hardships of the veteran's service, the veteran's lay testimony alone may establish the occurrence of the claimed in-service stressor."

Rebuttal 3: St. Petersburg VARO requested on August 24, 2001 that I detail my experiences in Vietnam. I replied by mid September 2001. I recounted many of the fire fights that became an every day event during my tour and when and how I was wounded.

Rebuttal 4:   A complete medical assessment by Dr. Henry Jones M.D. (Diplomat American Board of Psychiatry and Neurology) was submitted to the VARO on October 19, 2001. He detailed my diagnosis as Acute Post Traumatic Stress Disorder, Chronic Post Traumatic Stress Disorder, and Depressive Reaction Prolonged. His letter also points out that I have been under his care since March 1997. 38 CFR §3.157(b) (2) requires the VA to accept a *private physician or layman* evidence when establishing an effective date. The rule reads "The date of receipt of such evidence will be accepted when the evidence furnished by or in behalf of the claimant is within the competence of the physician or lay person and shows the reasonable probability of entitlement to benefits."

Rebuttal 5: Dr. Jones first communicated on my behalf on October 19, 2001 not on 01-23-02 as alleged in the April 30 rating decision. Dr. Jones provided the VARO with a second assessment on August 19, 2002. This letter was in response to the VA request for medical treatment evidence on June 26, 2002. His second reply only confirmed his diagnosis of chronic PTSD.

Issue 2. Effective date of benefits

Statement: "Service connection for Post Traumatic Stress Disorder has been established with an evaluation of 70 percent effective January 23, 2002."

Rebuttal 1: On February 28, 2001 I filed notice to amend my original claim to include PTSD. Six months later (August 24, 2001) the VARO sent me a letter outlining what evidence was necessary to pursue the claim. Because I didn't know the difference between a formal claim and an informal claim, my notice of February 28, 2001 failed to clearly express what I wanted. I clarified this however on September 3, 2001, when I responded to the VA letter August 24, 2001. I was not advised by the VARO that I could not change the intent of my February 28, 2001 letter. This response was within the one year statutory limit. The purpose was to allow me sufficient time to obtain all the necessary records to file a complete claim within the one year frame.

38 CFR §3.155 holds any communication or action, indicating an intent to apply for one or more benefits under the laws administered by the Department of Veterans Affairs, from a claimant may be considered an informal claim. Such informal claim must identify the benefit sought. Upon receipt of an informal claim, if a formal claim has not been filed, an application form will be forwarded to the claimant for execution. *If received within one year from the date it was sent to the claimant, it will be considered filed as of the date of receipt of the informal claim.*

Rebuttal 2: The VA failed to respond in a timely manner (6 months) to my notice to amend my original claim to include PTSD. They also failed to provide VA form 21-4138. Statement in Support of Claim as required by 38 CFR §3.150. The regulation states in part "Upon request made in person or in writing by any person applying for benefits under the laws administered by the Department of Veterans Affairs, the appropriate application form will be furnished."

Issue 3. Erroneous denial of PTSD benefits 01-15-02

Statement: The rating decision dated January 15, 2001 denied service connection for PTSD.

Rebuttal 1: The Rating Board erred when they rated and denied service connection benefits for PTSD and violated 38 CFR §3.159(b). Justifying the premature denial for service connection the rating authority stated "there was no evidence in the file to support any indication of treatment for any disability such as anxiety and insomnia." They carried this premise further by adding the records were totally silent for any nervous problems.

Rebuttal 2: In the claim file at the time this decision was made there were three documents which established sufficient evidence to rate and grant service connection for PTSD: One, my sworn statement of September 03, 2001 in which I related the hostile environment I faced each and every day and that I was wounded. Two, Dr. Jones's letter, dated October 19, 2001, confirmed the severity of my condition. And three, VA rating decision dated June 26, 1971 granted service connection for combat wounds.

Rebuttal 3: The rating authority violated 38 CFR §3.102 when rating board member stated "the rule regarding benefits of reasonable doubt does not apply because the preponderance of evidence is unfavorable." The Court has stated the VA must tell exactly what evidence was superior to mine and Dr. Jones's sworn statements.

Rebuttal 4: The rating authority failed to explain why they did not consider the evidence of record in the file which was favorable to my claim. Case law established 13 years ago (10-12-90) in *Gilbert v. Derwinski* 1 VetApp.49 (1990) that the VA is mandated to explain its reasons or bases to the veteran and to the court its factual finding and its conclusion why the veteran was not entitled to the Benefit of Doubt. It can not simply say "a preponderance of evidence is unfavorable."

Issue 4. Benefits awarded as a single veteran

Statement: "We are paying you as a single veteran."

Rebuttal 1: Under 38 CFR §3.205(7) my award should have been granted as a married veteran with a spouse. Paragraph 7 of the regulation states "Any other secondary evidence which reasonably supports a belief by the Adjudicating activity that a valid marriage actually occurred is acceptable." This test was met when my wife and I both submitted sworn statements before a notary on February 19, 2002. In our statements we stated that we were married on March 21, 1971, San Antonio, Texas.

JUNE 25, 2003: VA OFFERS DECISION REVIEW OFFICERS SERVICES

In June 2003, the VA offered David Raz the option of choosing to have a Decision Review Officer (DRO) assigned to his case or proceeding with the appeals process. There are times when the service of a DRO will definitely work to your advantage. We felt very strongly that our case would win on appeal, so we had everything to gain and nothing to lose by requesting a local hearing. Convincing the local RO that we were entitled and able to prove it, it was more likely than not that the appeal would not be certified to the Board of Veterans Appeals (BVA) in Washington. Winning locally saved us between one and two years additional wait time. A copy of their letter (figure 3.16) is provided to acquaint you with the mechanics of what the Decision Review Officer (DRO) duties are. DROs are senior adjudicators who are picked at random from the DRO pool. They are supposed to review all of the relevant records, not just those from the last action.

	Fig. 3.16

DEPARTMENT OF VETERANS AFFAIRS
St. Petersburg Regional Office
P.O. BOX 1431
St. Petersburg FL 33731

JUNE 25, 2003

David Raz   In Reply Refer To: 317/APPEALS/MJM
909 Spruce Drive   C XX-XXX-887
Tampa, FL 34703   Raz, David

Dear Mr. Raz:

We received your written disagreement with the Department of Veterans Affairs (VA) decision of May 20, 2001. This letter describes what happens next.

We will try to resolve your disagreement

This local office of the VA will try to resolve your disagreement through the Post-Decision Review Process. As part of this process, you must decide how you would like us to handle your appeal. You may choose to have a Decision Review Officer (DRO) assigned to your case or to follow the traditional appeal process.

How does the Decision Review Officer Process work?

Complete review: The Decision Review Officer will review the materials in your VA claims folder, including evidence and arguments, and statements from your representative. This may lead the Decision Review Officer to request additional evidence from you, your doctor or some other source. You may be asked to participate in an informal conference with the Decision Review Officer to discuss your case.

New decision: The DRO will then make a new decision. You will be notified of the decision by letter or provided a Statement of the Case with instructions to continue your Appeal.

How does the Traditional Appeal Process work?

Complete review: A VA staff member will check your file for completeness. Then a review will be made of your evidence and arguments, statements from your representative (if one has been designated) and any other information available in your claims folder, this may lead to a request for additional evidence from you, your doctor or other sources. You may be asked to clarify questions about your disagreement.

Statement of the Case: The reviewer will then prepare a Statement of Case (SOC) and send you a copy. The SOC will include a summary of the evidence, a citation to pertinent laws, a discussion of how those laws affect the decision, and a summary of the reasons for the decision. If you still do not agree with that decision and wish to continue your appeal, you need to submit a substantive appeal so that your case can be sent to the Board of Veterans' Appeals. Instructions on how to file a substantive appeal will be provided in our letter notifying you of the decision.

You may be Represented

You designated the American Legion to represent you in presenting your claim to VA. The Decision Review Officer will work with this representative while trying to resolve your disagreement. If you have not already done so, you should contact your representative directly to discuss your case.

How do I select the Decision Review Officer or Traditional Appeal Process?

You must notify us within 60 days from the date of this letter whether you want to have your case reviewed by the Decision Review Officer or by the traditional appeal process. If we do not hear from you within 60 days, your case will be reviewed under the traditional appeal process.

We hope we will be able to resolve your disagreement to your satisfaction. If you have questions about the information in this letter or any other aspect of your appeal, we encourage you to contact your accredited representatives if you have appointed one, or call our toll free telephone number 1-800-827-1000.

Sincerely yours,

B.O. Gibb
Veterans Service Center Manager

JULY 13, 2003: VETERAN ACCEPTS A DRO REVIEW

Figure 3.17 shows David's "Statement in Support of Claim," sent to the VA in July 2003. In responding to the VA's letter, state your case as you see it, based on the facts and regulations. When reviewing your response and the evidence of record, raters are required to give a detailed explanation as to why they continue to deny the claim. Once you have their brief (Statement of the Case), you can review it piece by piece using their regulations, manuals, general counsel opinions, and case law.

David Raz notified VA, within the sixty-day suspense period, that he was requesting his Notice of Disagreement be reviewed by a Decision Review Officer at RO. Included was a four-page timeline of key events and six questions the DRO must cover when deciding the merits of the NOD. The six questions were designed to keep the DRO focused on the issues favorable to the vet.

Fig. 3.17

0MB Approved No. 2900-0075 Respondent Burden: 15 minutes

Department of Veterans Affairs   STATEMENT IN SUPPORT OF CLAIM

PRIVACY ACT INFORMATION: The law authorizes us to request the information we are asking you to provide on this form (38 U.S.C. 501(a)) and (b)). The responses you submit are considered confidential (38 U.S.C. 5701). They may be disclosed outside the Department of Veterans Affairs (VA) only if the disclosure is authorized under the Privacy Act, including the routine uses identified in the VA system of records, 58VA21/22, Compensation, Pension, Education and Rehabilitation Records–VA, published in the Federal Register. The requested information is considered relevant and necessary to determine maximum benefits under the law. Information submitted is subject to verification through computer matching programs with other agencies.

RESPONDENT BURDEN: Public reporting burden for this collection of information is estimated to average 15 minutes per response, including the time for reviewing instructions, searching existing data sources, gathering and maintaining the data needed, and completing and reviewing the collection of information. Send comments regarding this burden estimate or any other aspect of this collection of information, including suggestions for reducing this burden, to the Clearance Officer (723), 810 Vermont Ave., NW, Washington, DC 20420; and to the Office of Management and Budget, Paperwork Reduction Project (2900-0057), Washington, DC 20503. PLEASE DO NOT SEND THIS FORM OR APPLICATION FOR BENEFITS TO THESE ADDRESSES.

FIRST NAME - MIDDLE NAME - LAST NAME OF VETERAN	SOCIAL SECURITY NO	VA FILE NO.
David F Raz	XXX-XX-7777	CXX-XXX-889

The following statement is made in connection with a claim for benefits in the case of above-named veteran:

In response to your letter of June 25, 2003 I elect to have a Decision Review Officer (DRO) assigned to my case. Attached is a four page summary of events I want the DRO to consider when deciding on the merits of my notice of disagreement. Should the DRO not reverse the rating board decision of 01-15-02 then the six questions posed on pages 3 & 4 of this attachment should be answered in detail. The Statement of the Case should not include statement such as "The rule of reasonable doubt does not apply because the preponderance of evidence is unfavorable" without a full explanation of what evidence is superior to my evidence and why it is superior. I also want you to cite the CFRs and case law that support your position.

I CERTIFY THAT the statements on this form are true and correct to best of my knowledge

SIGNATURE   **DATE**
SIGNED
David Raz
July 13, 2003

ADDRESS   **TELEPHONE NUMBERS**
909 Spruce Drive, Tampa, Florida 34703   **727-555-1212   None**

PENALTY The law provides severe penalties which Include fine or imprisonment or both, for the willful submission of any statement or evidence of a material fact, knowing it to be false.

VA FORM 21-4138 JUN 2000   21-4138
APR 994, WILL BE USED

01-28-02 VA letter states they rated claim for PTSD and denied the Benefits. Reason no Evidence in claim file.

02-19-02 VA Form 21-4138 submitted disagreeing with the 01-28-02 denial of benefits. Restated that VA advised on 09-03-01 that Informal claim was filed 02-28-01. Attached sworn statement of self, wife, and a letter of evaluation by Dr. Jones.

04-09-02 VA letter states working on pending claim.

06-26-02 VA sent Dr. Jones a letter requesting medical evidence on David. They gave a suspense date of 08-26-02 to respond.

08-19-02   Dr. Jones responds to VA request for detailed evaluation of David's PTSD condition. Response dated one week prior to 60 day suspense date.

09-09-02 VAMC send letter scheduling C&P Exam for PTSD on

09-24-02 VA states that they received Notice of Disagreement with their decision of 02-19-02 and that they were proceeding with the appeal process.

2003

04-30-03 VA advised that service-connection for PTSD was approved effective 02-01-02 and rated 70% disabling. Rating Board considered only evidence dated between 01-23-02 and 09-16-02 without explaining why records of between 02-28-01 and 10-19-01 were not considered relevant to support an entitlement date of 02-28-01.

05-31-03 Notice of Disagreement filed challenging the effective date of 02-01-02 for service-connection for PTSD.

06-25-03 Letter from VA requesting whether the veteran will accept a Decision Review Officers reviewing his disagreement concerning the entitlement date of his service-connected for PTSD.

07-14-03 Veteran notified VA, within the 60 day suspense period, that he is requesting his Notice of Disagreement be review by a Decision Review Officer at RO. Also, he attached a three-page summary of key dates pertinent to entitlement date for benefits.

Part IV: 2004

APRIL 5, 2004: VA GRANTS NEW EFFECTIVE DATE
The decision letter from the DRO can be found in figure 3.18. By acknowledging that the effective date of the veteran's entitlement was one year earlier, the case was able to advance to the next level. The VA claim reviewers resolved the issue by changing the effective date of entitlement to March 1, 2001. By forcing the issue, the veteran obtained an additional $13,000 in benefits from the VA.

However, Sgt. David Raz is still in limbo because he is not considered eligible for increased benefits because of unemployability. In stating the veteran's disability was 70% in 2001, they should have automatically considered him for Total Disability based on Individual Unemployability at a 100% rate. They did not do this. A formal claim was initiated July 9, 2004, for TDIU benefits.

January 2002 was the forty-sixth month since Sergeant Raz applied for compensation benefits based on PTSD. The battle is still not over. If the past is any indication, it may be 2008 before a conclusion is reached on this man's entitlements.

Fig. 3.18

DEPARTMENT OF VETERANS AFFAIRS
RO 317
PO BOX 1437
ST. PETERSBURG, FL 33731

David Raz

VA File Number
XX XXX-889

Represented by:
AMERICAN LEGION

Decision Review Officer Decision
March 23, 2004

INTRODUCTION

You performed honorable active service from March 13, 1969 to December 19, 1970 in the US Army. We received your Notice of Disagreement on June 10, 2003 with one or more of our earlier decisions. You requested a *denovo* review of your claim. A *denovo* review is a review of the claims file as permitted under the provisions of 38 CFR 3.2600. This review incorporates all the evidence of record, and is a new and complete review without deference to any prior determination.

Based on a review of the evidence listed below, we have made following decision(s) on your claim.

DECISION

Service connection for post traumatic stress disorder is established effective March 1, 2001.

EVIDENCE

Claims file review to include:
   •Statement February 28, 2001 from the veteran
          Statements dated January 23, 2002 and August 19, 2002, Dr. Jones
   •Examination September 16, 2002, VAMC Bay Pines

REASONS FOR DECISION

Evaluation of post traumatic stress disorder, competent currently evaluated as 70 percent disabling.

Service connection for post traumatic stress disorder requires medical evidence establishing a clear diagnosis of the condition, and credible supporting evidence that the claimed in-service stressor actually occurred, and a link, established by medical evidence, between current symptomatology and the claimed in-service stressor. A diagnosis of post traumatic stress disorder must meet all diagnostic criteria as stated in the *Diagnostic and Statistical Manual of Mental Disorders DSM-IV* published by the American Psychiatric Association.

On March 1, 2001, we received your initial claim for compensation for post traumatic stress disorder. Coincident with this claim, we obtained medical evidence, particularly reports from Dr. Jones, showing you have been undergoing treatment since March 1997 for psychiatric symptoms now diagnosed as post traumatic stress disorder. The claim was initially denied by rating action January 15, 2002, with which you timely submitted a formal Notice of Disagreement. Based on the evidence contained in your claims file, we determined that your psychoneurosis, now diagnosed as post traumatic stress disorder, is related to your military service. Service connection is, therefore, warranted.

Rating action April 30, 2003 granted service connection effective January 23, 2002 the date of Dr. Jones letter received on February 19, 2002. This rating action failed to properly apply the provisions of 38 CFR 3.156 and 38 CFR 3.400(b).

Corrective action is taken hereunder.

Service connection for post traumatic stress disorder is established effective March 1, 2001. An evaluation of 70 percent is assigned from March 1, 2001. The effective date of entitlement is the date of your claim and represents the earliest date from which benefits are payable under 38 CFR 3.156 and 38 CFR 3.400(b)(2).

Since there is a likelihood of improvement, the assigned evaluation is not considered permanent and is subject to a future review examination.*

REFERENCES:

Title 38 of the Code of Federal Regulations, Pensions, Bonuses and Veterans' Relief contains the regulations of the Department of Veterans Affairs which govern entitlement to all veteran benefits. For additional information regarding applicable laws and regulations, please consult your local library.

---

*   The *denovo* review was a fair and careful review until the last paragraph when the reviewer made an assumption that was contrary to evidence in the file. The paragraph is quoted to illustrate the point: "Since there is a likelihood of improvement, the assigned evaluation is not considered permanent and is subject to a future review examination." Yet there is no evidence in the file that suggests the condition of a veteran with PTSD will improve. By failing to make the initial rating permanent, the VA has made it possible to recall the veteran for additional C&P examinations and to review his evaluation.

JUNE 22, 2004: VETERAN SUBMITS FORMAL APPLICATION FOR TDIU BENEFITS

Sergeant Raz filed a formal application (VA Form 21-8940) for increased benefits owing to unemployability. It would be easy for the veteran to overlook this notice among a considerable collection of miscellaneous sheets of information attached to the VA letters. It is very important to submit the prescribed form when it is your intent to apply for Total Disability based on Individual Unemployability. This notice of possible entitlement was attached to the schedule of monthly benefit payments.

There are certain circumstances in which the VA should initiate development of a TDIU before the form is submitted. When a medical report received from a physician indicates the veteran's condition is chronic and permanent and that he is unemployable because of his PTSD, the rater must accept this as an informal claim on behalf of the veteran. The U.S. Court of Appeals for the Federal Circuit held in *Moody v. Principi*[5]: the "VA is to fully and sympathetically develop the veterans claim to its optimum before deciding its merits." This was not the case for Sergeant Raz.

JULY 9, 2004: VETERAN NOTIFIES VA OF FAILURE TO CONSIDER TDIU

The notice in figure 3.19 tells the VA raters that they should have notified the veteran that an informal claim of 100% for TDIU was established by Dr. Jones's letter dated October 19, 2001. This letter provided a foundation on which to claim that the veteran's condition was so severe that he was rated 70% disabled. When a veteran is disabled to the extent that his service-connected disability prevents him from being employed, the law says he shall be granted an 100% rating owing to unemployability.

Fig. 3.19

OMB Approved No. 2900-0075 Respondent Burden: 15 minutes

Department of Veterans Affairs   STATEMENT IN SUPPORT OF CLAIM

PRIVACY ACT INFORMATION: The law authorizes us to request the information we are asking you to provide on this form (38 U.S.C. 501(a)) and (b)). The responses you submit are considered confidential (38 U.S.C. 5701). They may be disclosed outside the Department of Veterans Affairs (VA) only if the disclosure is authorized under the Privacy Act, including the routine uses identified in the VA system of records, 58VA21/22, Compensation, Pension, Education and Rehabilitation Records–VA, published in the Federal Register. The requested information is considered relevant and necessary to determine maximum benefits under the law. Information submitted is subject to verification through computer matching programs with other agencies.

RESPONDENT BURDEN: Public reporting burden for this collection of information is estimated to average 15 minutes per response, including the time for reviewing instructions, searching existing data sources, gathering and maintaining the data needed, and completing and reviewing the collection of information. Send comments regarding this burden estimate or any other aspect of this collection of information, including suggestions for reducing this burden, to the Clearance Officer (723), 810 Vermont Ave., NW, Washington, DC 20420; and to the Office of Management and Budget, Paperwork Reduction Project (2900-0057), Washington, DC 20503. PLEASE DO NOT SEND THIS FORM OR APPLICATION FOR BENEFITS TO THESE ADDRESSES.

FIRST NAME - MIDDLE NAME - LAST NAME OF VETERAN	SOCIAL SECURITY NO	VA FILE NO.
David F Raz	XXX-XX-7777	CXX-XXX-889

The following statement is made in connection with a claim for benefits in the case of above-named veteran:

In response to your letter of April 5, 2004 adjusting my service-connected PTSD rating to 70 percent effective March 1, 2001 you failed to consider an additional entitlement for Total Disability for Individual Unemployability (TDIU.)

Judge Green writing for the Court in *Robert Norris v. Togo D. West* (97-347) decided June 9,1999, that CFR Par 4.16 (c) directs the Secretary to award a rating of 100% for TDIU when mental disorders cause unemployability. The Court further stated in section 4.16(c) The Secretary is aware that the 70% "requirement of 4.16(c) may be superfluous in light of the fact that whenever unemployability is caused by a service-connected mental, disorder regardless of its current disability rating, a 100% scheduler rating is warranted under section 4.132. Therefore, section 4.16 is not a limiting provision but an additionally, encompassing provision albeit perhaps, superfluous. Actually, it may be deemed more procedural device than a regulation which confers substantive benefit."

I CERTIFY THAT the statements on this form are true and correct to best of my knowledge

SIGNATURE **David Raz**

DATE SIGNED **July 9, 2004**

ADDRESS 909 Spruce Drive, Tampa, Florida   34703
TELEPHONE NUMBERS 727-555-1212   None

PENALTY The law provides severe penalties which Include fine or imprisonment or both, for the willful submission of any statement or evidence of a material fact, knowing it to be false.

VA FORM 21-4138 JUN 2000   21-4138
APR 994, WILL BE USED

AUGUST 17, 2004: VA INITIATES DELAYING TACTIC

The VA responded to David's formal request for TDIU benefits by asking again for the same complete package of information and evidence sent in July 2004. The claim reviewers also advised they would do nothing on his claim for two months, pending his response. The letter also included an Expedited Action Attachment, which authorizes the VA to rate the claim without waiting the sixty days established by statute. The purpose of this sixty-day waiting period is to give the veteran two months to submit additional evidence before the claim is rated. The wavier was signed because our evidence package was already of record. A copy of the Expedited Action Attachment and the signed wavier, dated August 20, 2004, can be viewed in figure 3.20.

Fig. 3.20

File Number: **XX XXX 887**
David Raz
VETERAN/CLAIMANT NAME: David Raz   CLAIM NUMBER: *XX XXX7 887*

EXPEDITED ACTION ATTACHMENT

By law, VA must wait 60 days from the date of this letter before making a decision on your claim in order for you to submit additional evidence. However, if you have no further evidence to submit, you may request that we process your claim as soon as we are able, notwithstanding this 60-day time period.

Please note there are now two options to respond to this attachment. You may either return this form to our office or call us at 1-800-827-1000. When you call, please inform the Veterans Service Representative that you are calling in reference to the "Expedited Action Attachment." This will allow for the representative with whom you are speaking to take the appropriate actions to expedite the processing of your claim. Also, please have this attachment in your possession when calling as you will be asked to provide some information contained within this form.

In response to this Veterans Claims Assistance Act (VCAA) letter, I have no additional relevant medical evidence to submit and request that you take the next action in processing my claim. I realize that I have until *08/17/05*, which is one year after the date of VA letter dated *08/17/04* to submit additional evidence and protect my entitlement to benefits from the earliest possible date.

Signature of Veteran/Claimant **David Raz**

Date **August 20, 2004**

Please remember to sign this document before mailing it to our office.

SEPTEMBER 20, 2004: VETERAN SENDS FOLLOW-UP NOTICE

David Raz sent a follow-up notice to his signed Expedited Action Attachment letter dated August 20, 2004. The purpose was to ensure the VA raters knew they had all the evidence necessary to rate his claim.

SEPTEMBER 29, 2004: VA DENIES TDIU BENEFITS

Within ten days, the VA reviewed Sergeant Raz's claim for TDIU benefits and denied it on the grounds that he was employable and his condition was not considered permanent. The mail time to the VA, internal mail distribution time, and processing by the adjudication division (which includes evaluating all the evidence, preparing a denial letter, and dispatching it) added up to only thirty-two workdays from the date David Raz filed his claim for TDIU benefits. That is a record for any VA Regional Office. It is obvious the claim was denied without anyone looking at it. The first two pages of the denial letter are shown in figure 3.21.

Fig. 3.21

DEPARTMENT OF VETERANS AFFAIRS
ST. Petersburg VARO
P.O. Box 1437
St. Petersburg, FL 33731

David Raz

VA File Number C-XX XXX 889

Represented by:
AMERICAN LEGION

Rating Decision
September 29, 2004

INTRODUCTION

The records reflect that you are a veteran of the Vietnam Era. You served in the United States Army for the period March 13, 1969, to December 19. 1970. You filed a new claim for benefits that was received on August 9, 2004. Based on a review of the evidence listed below, we have made the following decision on your claim.

DECISION

Entitlement to Individual Unemployability (IU) is denied

EVIDENCE

- Notarized "Statement of Last Day Employed" from veteran dated June 22, 2004
- Notarized Employment Statement from Mr. John Landers dated July 28, 2004.
- VA Form 21-8940, *Veteran's Application for Increased Compensation Based on Unemployability* received on August 6, 2004.

REASONS FOR DECISION

Entitlement to Individual Unemployability (IU).

Entitlement to individual unemployability is denied because the claimant has not been found unable to secure or follow a substantially gainful occupation as a result of service-connected disabilities. The evidence of record reveals veteran is currently service connected for Post-Traumatic Stress Disorder (PTSD) - 70% and Shell Fragment Wound (SFW) Right Upper Eyelid and Left Scalp - 0%. Veteran's combined service-connected evaluation is 70% effective March 1, 2001, which meets the requirements for IU as outlined in 38 CFR 4.16(a).

Notarized "Statement of Last Day Employed" from veteran dated June 22, 2004 informs the VA that he last worked for the United States Post Office on September 18, 2002. After that date he was on extended sick leave until all his leave was used. He would then be officially retired on November 28, 2003.

Notarized Employment Statement from Mr. John Landers dated July 28, 2004 reveals that in July 2003, he hired veteran to work for him part-time. Veteran had difficulties with balance and would frequently fall off a small ladder. Often he would get excited and work too fast and cut himself doing simple tasks. The liability was too much. Veteran was employed part-time until November 2003, when it was impossible to have him work for [Mr. Landers] in any capacity.

On his VA Form 21-8940, *Veteran's Application for Increased Compensation Based on Unemployability* received on August 6, 2004; veteran indicated that he last worked full time on September 18, 2002, as a letter carrier with the United States Postal Service. It is further noted that veteran had tried to obtain employment on July 1, 2003, with "John Landers Home Maintenance, Co.", since he claimed to be too disabled to work. Education is shown as three (3) years of college with no additional training or education.

Upon reviewing above mentioned evidence and that in the Claims Folder it is noted that veteran has two (2) service-connected disabilities with a combined effective date of March 1, 2001. However, at this time veteran's claim must be denied because he has a pending Compensation and Pension Review Examination scheduled as his service connected PTSD has not been determined to be permanent.

REFERENCES

Title 38 of the Code of Federal Regulations, Pensions, Bonuses and Veterans' Relief contains the regulations of the Department of Veterans Affairs, which govern entitlement to all veteran benefits. For additional information regarding applicable laws and regulations, please consult yow local library, or visit us at our web site, www.va.gov.

OCTOBER 26, 2004: VETERAN TRIES TO VERIFY
DATE OF C&P EXAM

The denial letter dated September 29, 2004, referred to a pending C&P Exam due in September 2004. The question that jumps out of the denial letter is why would the VA rate a claim, knowing that new medical evidence might alter the rating?

The VA Medical Center Bay Pines was contacted and asked to check on what day the C&P Exam was scheduled. After typing the information into the computer, the clerk came back with an excuse she was having some trouble and would David call back in about an hour. The next time David talked to the clerk, later that day, she read off the computer that his appointment was scheduled for November 10, 2004. He would receive written conformation within a few days.

OCTOBER 2, 2004: MEDICAL CENTER CONFIRMS C&P EXAM

VA Medical Center Bay Pines confirmed the November 10, 2004, appointment. The failure of the RO to coordinate and follow up on the alleged September C&P Exam will be one of the appeal arguments should the veteran continue through the complete process to obtain his TDIU benefits.

OCTOBER 29, 2004: RO ALERTS VET PENDING C&P EXAM

Strangely, a letter from the RO arrived three days later advising that a required C&P review evaluation had been scheduled. If the veteran had not made that telephone call to inquire about this alleged September C&P Exam its doubtful if would have ever heard from the RO concerning an exam.

NOVEMBER 4, 2004: VETERAN FILES NOTICE OF DISAGREEMENT

Figure 3.22 is the response the veteran filed on November 4, 2004, rebutting the VA reasoning for denying his claim for TDIU. This is an example of a NOD that puts the VA raters on defense. They have to address every rebuttal point to explain why they ignored their own regulations, manuals, and court decisions. One of the best suggestions I can offer to anyone going head to head with the VA is to take the initiative. Demand answers to your questions or your challenges.

OMB Approved No. 2900-0075 Respondent Burden: 15 minutes

Fig. 3.22

Department of Veterans Affairs   STATEMENT IN SUPPORT OF CLAIM

PRIVACY ACT INFORMATION: The law authorizes us to request the information we are asking you to provide on this form (38 U.S.C. 501(a)) and (b)). The responses you submit are considered confidential (38 U.S.C. 5701). They may be disclosed outside the Department of Veterans Affairs (VA) only if the disclosure is authorized under the Privacy Act, including the routine uses identified in the VA system of records, 58VA21/22, Compensation, Pension, Education and Rehabilitation Records–VA, published in the Federal Register. The requested information is considered relevant and necessary to determine maximum benefits under the law. Information submitted is subject to verification through computer matching programs with other agencies.

RESPONDENT BURDEN: Public reporting burden for this collection of information is estimated to average 15 minutes per response, including the time for reviewing instructions, searching existing data sources, gathering and maintaining the data needed, and completing and reviewing the collection of information. Send comments regarding this burden estimate or any other aspect of this collection of information, including suggestions for reducing this burden, to the Clearance Officer (723), 810 Vermont Ave., NW, Washington, DC 20420; and to the Office of Management and Budget, Paperwork Reduction Project (2900-0057), Washington, DC 20503. PLEASE DO NOT SEND THIS FORM OR APPLICATION FOR BENEFITS TO THESE ADDRESSES.

FIRST NAME - MIDDLE NAME - LAST NAME OF VETERAN	SOCIAL SECURITY NO	VA FILE NO.
David F Raz	XXX-XX-7777	CXX-XXX-889

The following statement is made in connection with a claim for benefits in the case of above-named veteran:

In response to your letter of September 29, 2004 I hereby file a Notice of Disagreement in which *Individual Unemployability* was denied. Your letter of denial failed to give reasons and basis for the decision. It stated benefits were "denied because the claimant has not been found unable to secure or follow a substantially gainful occupation as a result of his service connected disabilities."

Rebuttal:
Paragraph 1. The rater stated that I have not shown that I could not secure substantial gainful occupation. First let's address the legal definition of <u>Substantial</u> and <u>Gainful Occupation</u> as define in *Black's Law Dictionary.* *

Substantial means "something worthwhile as distinguished from something without value or merely nominal."

I CERTIFY THAT the statements on this form are true and correct to die best of my knowledge and belief

SIGNATURE **David Raz**   DATE SIGNED **November 04, 2004**
ADDRESS   TELEPHONE NUMBERS (Include Area Code)
909 Spruce Street, Tampa FL 31703   DAYTIME   EVENING
                                         727-555-1212   Same

PENALTY: The law provides severe penalties which include fine or imprisonment, or both, for the willful submission of any statement or evidence of a material fact, knowing it to be false.

VA FORM	EXISTING STOCKS OF VA FORM 214138,
JUN 2000	21-4138APR 1994, WILL BE USED

Gainful Occupation means within a disability "as ordinary employment of a particular individual or other such employment, if any the individual may be expected to follow." (*Black's Law Dictionary 5th Edition* pages 610 & 1280 (1979)

Had the rater considered the definition in the context of the evidence in the claim file he would have to justify why he failed to take into consideration the statement of Dr. Henry Jones, Board Certified Psychiatrist evaluation of January 23, 2002 where he stated that not only was my **"condition chronic** but **permanent."** This diagnosis goes back to March 25, 1997 when Dr. Jones saw me on an emergency basis.

Within my claim file is a letter to the VA from Dr. Jones dated August 19, 2002 in which he states "even with medication, the stress of these situations that David has a tendency to 'bottle up' becomes to much and his Post Traumatic Stress Disorder disability once gain exacerbates, leaving him incapacitated. When he is incapacitated, even simple living tasks at home become hard for him to accomplish."

To this end the General Counsel Decision <u>VAOPGCPREC</u> <u>10-95</u> states the duration of symptoms necessary to establish chronic post-traumatic stress disorder has been changed from six months or more to three months or more.** *See* DSM-III at 238 and DSM-IV at 429.

"I have been dealing with PTSD for more than three decades and have been in continuous therapy with David for more than seven years."

Paragraph 3. The rater notes that I was no longer actively employed after September 18, 2002. He did not acknowledge that the reason for my absences was my PTSD disability. Altogether since 2001, I missed 70 weeks of work due to effects of PTSD. (Attached as supportive evidence is a copy of the Post Offices Absence Analysis.)

Paragraph 4. Mr. Landers's letter to the VA was given no probative consideration. His letter described the manner in which I performed my assigned tasks. The difficulty with balance and frequently falling off a small step ladder is indicative of the side effects associated with Ativan and Zoloft. (See attached Pharmaceutical Information concerning these two drugs.) The rater having supposedly reviewed the claim file should have consulted the Physicians Desk Reference to help evaluate the limitations imposed on any possible work environment due to these drugs. Employers will not employ anyone who must take controlled drugs because of the risk at the job site, increased premium cost for health insurance, increase cost for workman's compensation coverage, and they also know that the individual can not guarantee that he will come to work every day.

Paragraph 6. The rater held that the "claim must be denied" because I had a pending Compensation and Pension Review Evaluation scheduled [because] my service connection "has not been determined to be Permanent."

The C&P evaluation for PTSD for *Review Examination* was not known to me. A call to the C&P appointment desk at Bay Pines VA Medical Center revealed that an exam was scheduled for November 10, 2004. In view of the fact that it took the clerk one hour to tell me when the appointment was scheduled I'm concerned that if I had not called I might have never been scheduled. Therefore if my claim is not granted, under the provisions of the Freedom of Information Act I want a copy of the order requesting a review examination and a copy of the Medical Centers Response. The records show that I was given an initial C&P evaluation on September 16, 2002.

It must be noted that at every step of the way from the initial claim for benefits, to the correct effective date of entitlement and now the claim for TDIU benefits a Notice of Disagreement had to be initiated. From the style & form of the letter it is obvious that the claim file received a "Top Sheeting" review. The rater failed to follow not only the 38 CFR, M-21-1 but all associated case law by the United States Court of Appeals for Veterans Claims in arriving at his decision to deny benefits.

The Court ruled in *Gabrielson v. Brown 7 Vet.App 36, 39-40 (1994)* that the VA must analyze the credibility and probative value of the evidence, accounts for the evidence which it finds to be persuasive or unpersuasive, and provide the reasons for its rejection of any material favorable to the veteran. The rater of this claim completely ignored the Court's ruling in this case.

38 CFR §3.340 (a) Total and permanent total rating and Unemployability*

My claim meets the standards set forth in 38 CFR§ 3.340(a) in that there is no requirement for entitlement for PTSD disability to be rated permanent before TDIU benefits may be granted. Further, in the same paragraph it states "Total disability will be considered to exist when there is present any impairment of mind or body which is sufficient to render it impossible for the average person to follow a substantially gainful occupation.

When you incorporate the legal description of substantially and gainful employment the evidence in my file supports the awarding of TDIU benefits. The supporting evidence in my claim folder removes any doubt that my disability is chronic and permanent, I have been unable to work at any level of employment because stress caused by working under supervision and meeting assigned performance standards. As the record shows Dr, Jones advised the Regional Office on several occasions that (a) I need to be medicated for the rest of my life and (b) the instance of job stress will cause a full grown exacerbation leaving me totally incapacitated.

PTSD Case Review^{****}
In January 2001 the Director of for Compensation and Pension sent a memo to all Regional Officers and Centers relating the finding of a special review ordered by his office. Many of these points made nearly four years ago are repeated in the adjudication of my claim. Here is a short lists of procedural errors RO were told to correct in dealing with PTSD claims. However, in the adjudication of my claim they were ignored.

Problem in applying rating schedule criteria
One reason for erroneous valuations may be confusion about the criteria in the general rating formula for mental disorders. The signs and symptoms named at each level are examples of what might be seen at each level. However, the absence of those specific findings in an individual does not exclude a rating at any given level.

It is the described effects on social and occupational functioning at each level of whatever signs and symptoms the veteran has that should determine the rating. In particular, the examples of signs and symptoms given do not encompass the common diagnostic findings specific to *PTSD,* but apply to any mental disorder. Therefore, you must look beyond the generic signs and symptoms in the rating schedule and look at the effects of PTSD in that individual. As with other disabilities, there is often a difference between the findings that establish the diagnosis of PTSD and those that indicate its level of severity.

Example; Vietnam combat veteran reported or showed: sleep disturbances to point of getting only 3-4 hours of sleep a night, avoidance of most people and social events, distant and estranged from others, restricted range of affect, aggressive outbursts at work indicating impaired judgment in thinking (almost threw a man off a building, drove a vehicle into something else and caused damage), withdrawn, decreased concentration, hypervigilance, mood, depressed and hopeless, suicidal ideation, fatigued and irritable, hallucinatory flashbacks, impairment in reality testing.

Some of these are examples (in the general rating formula for mental disorders) of signs and symptoms at the 70% evaluation level, and others are more akin to the 100% level. Some of his significant problems are not in either list of examples. Taking into account all of the findings, it is clear he is at least severely, if not totally, impaired in social and occupational functioning. He was given a 70% evaluation. Others might judge a 100% evaluation as more appropriate, particularly in view of the episodes of violence.

The National PTSD Center points out that the presence of violence toward self and others in the veteran's history is a significant feature that should drop the GAF score into the lower ranges, even if functioning in other areas appears better. This indicates the Center's belief that violence should be regarded as an indication of very serious disease.

Reluctance to grant 100%
Reluctance to grant 100% many cases of PTSD were rated at 70% even when there were clear indications on the examination that the veteran had severe symptoms and had total occupational impairment because of PTSD symptoms.

Examples: One veteran had not been working for 2 years because of PTSD symptoms; one was reported as unable to work and getting progressively worse; one had not worked for 7 or 8 months since seeing "Saving Private Ryan"; one was complying with his treatment plan but was said not to be sufficiently stable (e.g., had suicidal ideation) to maintain competitive employment; one was said to have an inability to function in almost all areas; and one had impairment of reality testing, active flashbacks, depression, hopeless mood, etc.

Each of these was rated at 70% but could have been rated at 100%. G* scores in these cases ranged from 30 to 45. (30 was the lowest GAF score given for any case in this review.) Most were eventually given I.O., but there seemed to be great reluctance to grant a schedular 100% evaluation even when there was ample medical evidence of severe disability due to PTSD, and a clear indication of impaired functioning sufficient for a schedular 100% evaluation.

The old *Physicians Guide* stated in the chapter on mental disorders: "In the case of anxiety disorders, except for severe phobias, it is unusual for a person to be completely incapacitated." However, VA's National PTSD Center states that anxiety disorders, severe phobias, PTSD, OCD (obsessive-compulsive disorder), panic disorder (esp. with agoraphobia), and social phobia all can be debilitating, sometimes to the point of complete incapacitation. Currently, over 29,000 veterans with PTSD are rated at 100% and over 6,000 with generalized anxiety disorder are rated at 100%. Therefore, it is no longer correct to say that total incapacitation for anxiety disorders are unusual.

What problems were found on notification letters?

A common problem on notification noted in the review was the failure to provide correct and adequate notification letters. A letter notifying a claimant about a rating should not simply refer to rating for all information, only for a more detailed explanation of the notification letter itself. (See M21—1, Part III, 11.09a and FL 00-58.)

In Summary

Should the rating officer upon reviewing my rebuttal fail to grant me a 100% service connection for PTSD a Statement of the Case will be issued by him but, must address these issues:

- a. Why the rater believe that the evidence in my file does not profile the example of the Vietnam veteran used as an example by Director Epley in this letter criticizing RO's handling of PTSD cases. In his example the Director said 100% would be in order therefore, why are the facts in my case any less disabling than that veterans.
- b. Why the rater reasoned that TDIU could not be granted because it was not adjudicated as permanent. I want the response to cite the appropriate CFR, M-21-1 and case law that supports his decision.
- c. I want the rater to state exactly what his evidence is when analyzed, would establish that evidence favorable to me was not persuasive and creditable.
- d. Explain the reason why the evidence did not qualify for a favorable decision under the Doctrine of Reasonable doubt.
- e. Explain why that this is the third time it was necessary for me to appeal a decision before the claim was given a proper evaluation.
- f. Explain why the rater held he had to deny the claim because I was scheduled for a C&P Review in September 2004 when in fact no exam was ever scheduled until I called the C&P Center at Bay Pines.
- g. Explain why the claim was rated when the rater acknowledged that he knew an exam was going to be required. This violates 38 CFR.

List of exhibits substantiating this rebuttal:
1. *Black's Law Dictionary* – Definition of Substantial Gainful Occupation;
2. Dr. Jones's letter of January 23, 2002;
3. Dr. Jones's letter of August 19, 2002;
4. General Counsel Opinion dated March 31, 1995 Para 7;
5. Rating Decision of September 29, 2004 Para 3;
6. Postal Services; Absence Analysis Year 2001, and 2002 (New Evidence);
7. Sworn Statement of John Landers dated 4-28-2004;
8. 38 CFR 3.340 Para 3.340(b);
9. PTSD Case Review, Director Compensation and Pension Services.

Justifying why these specific exhibits are cited:
Exhibits 1 is to call the raters attention to legal definition when consideration the terms Substantial and gainfully employed;
Exhibits 2, 3, 5, & 7 are part of my claim file and are added to focus the raters attention to the evidence which is favorable to me.
Exhibit 4 clarifies what constitutes a Chronic Medical Condition as it relates to PTSD;
Exhibit 6 Supports my statement that I Missed 70 weeks of work between 2001 and 2003;
Exhibit 8   A pertinent CFR pertaining to PTSD;
Exhibit 9 Established that the Director of Compensation and Pension has instructed rating board members nearly 4 years ago what and how they are to rate PTSD claims. His letter supports my belief the claim was not properly adjudicated. I should have been granted 100% permanently at the time originally adjudicated.
Exhibit 10 C&P Examination PTSD 09-16, 2004;
Exhibit 11 Description and Use of Zoloft;
Exhibit 12 Description and Use of Ativan;
Exhibit 13 38 CFR 4.15 Total Disability Rating;
Exhibit 14 38 CFR 4.16 TD rating for compensation based on Unemployability of the individual;
Exhibit 15 38 CFR 4.18 Unemployability;
Exhibit 16 38 CFT 4.126 Evaluation of disabilities from mental disorders;
Exhibit 17 Global Assessment of Function Scale DSM –IV Axis V.

*   Pages 610 and 1020 from *Black's Law Dictionary* were copied and attached to his Notice of Disagreement. The purpose of this is to constrain the rater's interpretation of what constitutes "substantial and gainful occupation." It is important to remember that the person rating your claim is not necessarily right and all knowing. Rating board members do not have legal or medical training.

**   General counsel opinions are very important and are binding on rating board members. If you find where the adjudicator ignored a GC opinion, you have a winning hand. To find opinions on the Internet, use Google to search for the term "VAOPGCREC 10-95."

***   Code of Federal Regulations, title 38, 3.340 governs *total and permanent total ratings and unemployability* and is the authority to grant a 100% rating.

****   The director of the Compensation and Pension Administration ordered a PTSD case review. The results didn't favor the veteran suffering from PTSD. To read the entire report, point your browser to http://obama.senate.gov/press 050810_obama_criticizes_va_decision_to_review_72000_post_traumatic_stress_disorder_cases/index.html.

NOVEMBER 12, 2004: NURSE PRACTITIONER CONDUCTS REVIEW EXAMINATION FOR PTSD

A nurse practitioner conducted the C&P evaluation without the supervision of a board-certified psychiatrist. The use of a nurse practitioner in place of a doctor to perform a C&P examination raises questions as to the thoroughness of the examination. The margin for errors increases tenfold when decisions are delegated to the inexperienced medical staff members. The VA procedures allow for review examinations to be performed by others besides doctors to justify claim denials. A copy of the report forwarded to the St. Petersburg Regional Office can be viewed in figure 3.23.

If the RO refuses to grant TDIU benefits, we will attack the report as "flawed" because of its deviation from the protocol format. In this case the examiner failed to express the opinion that David's condition was permanent and will not improve. He also failed to address the employability factor.

	Fig. 3.23

Progress Note

TITLE:C&P EXAMINATION

DATE OF NOTE: NOV 10, 2004@11:00

ENTRY DATE: NOV 12, 2004@09:32:06

AUTHOR: ROBERTS, DAVID   EXP COSIGNER:

URGENCY: STATUS: CONFLETED

SUBJECT: 99999

PATIENT NAME: RAZ, DAVID

Review examination for post traumatic stress disorder.

This is a 61-year-old gentleman. C-file was reviewed. He is 70% service connected for post traumatic stress disorder and this is a review examination. He has no record of being treated here. He is seen by a private psychiatrist. He was seen for years by Dr. Jones in the private sector and currently by Dr. Smith since Dr. Jones retired. He is being treated for post traumatic stress disorder with Zoloft 103 mg half a tablet four times a day and lorazepam 0.5 mg four times a day. For reference, there is a letter in the C-File dated August 19, 2002, from Dr. Jones which is quite informative. This patient's symptoms have been chronic with no remission. He reports increased anxiety. He no longer can do woodworking. He is more abrupt with his wife, more irritable, just generally finding himself more anxious and unable to do the things he enjoys and also increased depression. He last worked in November 2003. He retired from the Post Office. The last year and a half of that time was sick leave prior to retirement due to his symptoms from post traumatic stress disorder. He states he also had a nervous breakdown in 1995 and was out a considerable amount of time at that time. He has no social life. He has no friends. He denies all substance abuse.

MENTAL STATUS EXAMINATION:

There is no impairment of thought process or communication. He is not psychotic. Eye contact was good. There was no inappropriate behavior noted. There is occasional suicidal ideation with no plan or intent and no homicidal ideation since on medication. Hygiene is good and he does attend to his basic activities of daily living appropriately. He is oriented to person, place and time. He does indicate some short term memory deficit which I would relate to his depression which he rates 7-8 out of 0-10 and anxiety 9 out of 0-10. At these levels, his ability to focus and concentrate is impaired, thus adversely affecting his short term memory. There is no obsessive ritualistic behavior other than some Hypervigilance at night. Speech is fluent and relevant. He denies panic, but does avoid crowds for that reason. Impulse control is good. He sleeps about seven to eight hours, but does have bad dreams of Vietnam about every other month. He is competent for VA benefits. There are no other multiple mental disorder symptoms.

DIAGNOSIS:

AXIS I: Post traumatic stress disorder chronic, symptomatic.
AXIS II: Deterred.
AXIS III: Hyperlipidemia.
AXIS IV: Combat trauma.
AXIS V: GAF score of 50 with serious impairment in social and occupational
         functioning, no friends, social isolation, and occasional suicidal ideation.

   Dr. Johnson will be reviewing this examination.

   DD: 11/10/04   DT: 11/11/04   job: 999999   DR/ABC

   /es/ DAVID ROBERTS, ARNP

   ARNP-C&P

Signed: 11/16/2004 10:01

PATIENT NAME AND ADDRESS (Mechanical imprinting, if available VISTA Electronic Medical Documentation)

RAZ DAVID
909 SPRUCE DR
TAMPA FLORIDA 34703-1212   Printed at BAY PINES VAMC

DECEMBER 14, 2004: VA CONTINUES RATING AT 70%
Based on the C&P examination dated November 14, 2004, the VA has determined that David's PTSD remains 70% disabling. On the last page in the lower corner of the of the rating decision was the remark, "Individual Unemployability Denied." When David called to clarify the statement concerning the status of his appeal, he was advised the appeal had not been decided.

Part V: 2005

Another year will begin before Sergeant Raz is informed by the St. Petersburg Regional Office whether benefits will be conceded without any further action or whether a full-blown appeal will be necessary. It is my prediction that a resolution of David's claim will take several more years. The local RO doesn't want to go on record granting 100% for PTSD. They also don't want to be looked upon by the Central Office in Washington as the RO who gave $50,000 or more for a PTSD claim the first time it was reviewed. If the RO's decision is reversed by the Board of Veterans' Appeals and told to grant the benefits, the RO will be able to say, "We didn't grant the benefit; we were told to grant it by the BVA."

Chapter 3: What Have We Learned?

1. PTSD is not a newly identified medical phenomenon. Historical medical stories identified this disorder more than 2,700 years ago.
2. It took eight years after medical standard for PTSD was accepted by the medical profession before the VA was forced to deal with the issue of PTSD on a more realistic level.
3. The fourth version of *DSM* has redefined how long symptoms must exist before the condition is considered chronic. The new standard is three months.
4. Veterans who were tagged by the DOD or VA as having a personality disorder, compulsive disorder, paranoid disorder, or schizophrenia, and now have been diagnosed with PTSD should reopen their original claim for service connection.
5. Use Sergeant Raz outline of his dealing with the VA as a model for developing your claim for PTSD benefits. Later chapters will help you put your claim together so benefits are granted.
6. Sergeant Raz's case demonstrates the tenacity that is necessary to pursue your interest in having a claim approved. Don't believe the concept that a veteran dealing with the VA is an act of non-advocacy. The moment the claim is denied, that us versus them relationship is dissolved. Through a series of administrative steps, the parties enter the arena of civil legation.
7. Know the type of claim you are filing. For example if you have never filed a

claim with the VA, then you should file an original claim on form VA 21-526. Chapter 6 will tell you all about the various claim actions for filing a claim for PTSD.

8. Make certain you have proof that you are currently disabled by PTSD. It is preferable to be evaluated by a professional specialist who is willing to prepare a written assessment of your disability.

9. Prepare a time line of events as you remember them, using the time line Sergeant Raz submitted as a guide.

10. If you were wounded and received the Purple Heart, make sure it is stated on your discharge certificate (DD-214). The same is true with the Bronze Star. Send a copy of the award letter along with your application for benefits.

11. Make certain any statement you, your family, or your friends submits is sworn before a notary public.

12. If you have a valid claim, don't let the VA deny benefits. Remember Sergeant Raz has challenged raters on three occasions and two were victories for him and the third is pending. Remember! If you are turned down, appeal the denial.

13. The VA is not all knowing and the decisions from the local Regional Offices are not cast in cement, as we have demonstrated in this chapter.

14. Know where you can find their laws, regulations, opinions, and case law that support your claim.

Notes

1. Timeline submitted to the VA focusing on key dates and evidence supporting Sergeant Raz's PTSD claim. Submitting a timeline is a valuable technique to use. It forces the VA to look at evidence that favors you.

2. This is the initial notice to the VA that the veteran wanted to claim service connection for PTSD. See chapter 5 for the details concerning the various kinds of claims.

3. Dr. Jones's letter to the VA is an excellent example of how a doctor's statement supporting your claim for PTSD should be prepared. Remind the doctor when he is preparing a statement that the VA readers have no medical training; a letter written as if to a professional colleague would heighten the odds of having the claim denied. One other point of great importance: provide the doctor with a copy of 38 CFR Part IV, "Schedule for Rating Disabilities Section," Section 9400, when he states the degree disability resulting from PTSD. Also provide him with C&P examination: Initial or Review Examination for Post-Traumatic Stress Disorder (PTSD).

4. This is an example of the VA failing to follow its own regulations by rating the claim eight months prior to end date.

5. *Moody v. Principi*, 360 F. 1303 (3d. Cir. 2004).

Disability Claims Processing

In order to have your claim for PTSD benefits accepted, you must understand the rules and regulations of the VA and claims process. First, you need intelligence as to how a Regional Office is structured and operated. Believe me, fighting an enemy blind is no different than putting your faith in a giant bureaucracy such as the VA and expecting results automatically in your favor.

The Department of Veterans Affairs is administered through a network of fifty-seven VA Regional Offices. Disability compensation benefits covering chronic illnesses or injuries are one of the most expensive operational costs for the Department of Veterans Affairs.

The VA published a fact sheet in December 2004 titled "VA Disability Claims Processing." As you can see in figure 4.1, the text is biased in emphasizing how the VA is resolving operational problems benefiting veterans. Congressional representatives put pressure on the secretary of the Department of Veterans Affairs by passing several legislative acts that mandated reform.

Fig. 4.1

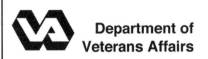

Office of Public Affairs   Washington, DC 20420
Media Relations   (202) 273-6000
                           www.va.gov

Department of Veterans Affairs | **Fact Sheet**

March 2005

VA Disability Claims Processing

The Department of Veterans Affairs (VA) fulfills the government's obligation to help those who leave the military injured or ill. In service to their country, military members give up the right to decline dangerous assignments. Their occupations lack conventional workers compensation coverage.

Administered through a network of 57 VA regional offices, disability compensation benefits cover chronic illnesses or injuries incurred during or worsened by military service. It is one of the VA's most extensive benefits and among the most complex, posing a challenge to timely service.

Current payment rates and background on the basis for determining the severity of a disability are available at http://www.va.gov/OPA/fact/05comprates.asp.

In fiscal year 2004, more than 703,000 veterans received decisions on their disability claims, and an additional 752,800 beneficiaries received decisions on claims not requiring a rating decision. VA added approximately 62,000 beneficiaries to its compensation and pension rolls, bringing the total number of beneficiaries of VA compensation and pension to nearly 3.5 million. Compensation and pension payments last year exceeded $30 billion.

VA has made a commitment to keeping its rating claims inventory to 250,000 claims with an average processing time of 145 days. As recently as 2002, VA had more than 432,000 disability claims pending and a processing time in excess of 233 days. A September 2003 decision by the Federal Circuit Court significantly affected both workload and the timeliness of VA decisions in 2004. The decision held that denial of a claim is premature before the expiration of the one-year period established by the Veterans Claims Assistance Act of 2000. As a result, decisions on more than 62,000 claims were deferred, many for as much as 90 days or longer. A provision of the Veterans Benefits Act of 2003 subsequently allowed VA to issue decisions on all of those cases deferred. VA's disability claims inventory is currently approximately 336,000, and the timeliness of completed claims is once again declining with average processing speed at 171 days. The inventory is also affected by an increasing volume of claims from veterans who served in Iraq and Afghanistan.

Claims Processing Improvement Task Force Spur Reforms

In response to a growing backlog of disability claims, coupled with an increasing number of days required to render a decision, VA commissioned a task force to study the processing methods and other performance drivers within the Veterans Benefits Administration and to make recommendations for corrective action. The Claims Processing Improvement Task Force made a number of recommendations early in fiscal year 2002. Key was the recommendation to shift the work processing method from the case management concept to that of the claims process improvement (CPI) model. The CPI model changed the manner in which claims are processed.

The CPI model differs from the case management model in a number of ways. For one thing, the CPI model allows for specialization of processing through the use of six specialized teams. Four of these teams address specific, critical cycles in claims processing: triage, pre-determination, rating, and post-determination. Two additional teams address important areas related to the process itself: Public Contact and Appeals. By shifting from an individual focus to a process focus, a number of improvements were gained. First, it became easier to spot process or flow disruptions since the work was organized around process flow and not individual assignments. Second, training and development could be very specific and focused. Third, the tools to monitor inventory were more effective in a process environment versus a case managed environment.

The Claims Processing Improvement Task Force also made a significant number of additional recommendations, the majority of which have been implemented. Additional information is available at http://www.va.gov/opa/fact/claimstf. Taken together, these recommendations created an integrated performance management system that not only complements the CPI model but has greatly enhanced the outcome.

Accountability, Performance Management Key to Reforms

The concept of accountability was a hallmark of the Task Force report. The specific methods used to convert the accountability concept to reality were in four linked areas.

- First, performance became a factor in resource allocation. Prior to CPI, resource allocation was based upon expected workload as well as other factors generally related to the existing inventory. The new Resource Allocation Model provides more resources to those offices that demonstrate sustained high performance and increased productivity. This would ultimately be a large driver for those offices achieving very high performance.

- Second, the prior method of annual office evaluations was abandoned in favor of very detailed monthly targets for VA regional offices. These targets covered a vast array of performance measures including output, inventory, quality, older cases, and two measures for timeliness (a leading indicator and a lagging indicator). Offices were tracked each month with respect to progress toward meeting these targets. Focus on these targets became a significant driver in improving performance.

- Third, these targets were integrated into the performance plans of each VA Regional Office director. This linkage of resources and clear expectations with a rapid feedback cycle for results had a dramatic affect on performance, particularly rating output.
- Fourth, VA developed a sophisticated reward and recognition system with three levels of recognition. High performing offices could receive significant award money for performing at levels well above the national averages. A study by a VA team reviewing cycle time in VA has looked at the impact of these performance drivers in VA and concluded that they are making a significant difference.

There were two other drivers of performance that worked in concert with the integrated performance management system. These also had their genesis in the recommendations from the Task Force. The first involved dynamic brokering of claim work from offices unable to keep pace to offices with excess capacity or to teams specifically developed to work bordered cases. VA developed both a network of resource centers, teams within certain offices whose mission was to work brokered cases, and a Tiger Team dedicated to processing cases involving older veterans whose claims had been pending more than one year.

VA developed a number of automated tools specifically aimed at improving process cycle times. These include the Inventory Management system, the Modern Award Processing-Development tool, and a number of specific reports generated weekly and monthly that allow VA Central Office and field managers to monitor progress toward goals as well as spot cycle time delays in time to take corrective actions.

# # #

Several sections in the fact sheet need to be reviewed from an impartial perspective. First, let's take a look at the figures presented in paragraph three. The VA notified 827,000 veterans of the results of their disability claims. In the next sentence, the VA announced that 256,000 compensation and pension claims were added to the rolls. Their statement is silent as to how many claims were granted for compensation or how many for pension. What they didn't present was how many of the 571,000 claims were denied. This tells us the best guess for determining causality rate is seven out of every ten claims is denied. It would be safe to assume that of the remaining three out of ten claims approved, one and a half to two would be for pension benefits.

The second issue raised by the fact sheet is how well claims are evaluated if there are more than 324,000 claims pending and the overall incentive for acceptable performance is based on how many claims can be processed per day. If in fact merit pay increases are tied to daily production, it is in the claims examiner's best interest to save time and deny claims when there isn't absolute proof easily understood by case-workers with no knowledge of complex medical or legal issues.

The hidden pressure forcing the VA to change the way it does business comes from the White House and the Office of Management and Budget (OMB).

If we are to assume that OMB executives dictate the amount of money spent on PTSD claims, evidence shows that the VA has been directed to deny claims whenever possible. It is even possible that in a meeting between the secretary of the Department of Veterans Affairs and the direct of OMB could have occurred stating this in no uncertain terms:

OMB director: "I don't care what you publicly tell veterans. Just do not give away the store for all these PTSD claims. It's bad enough we had to tiptoe around the congressional mandate in 1989 concerning supporting veterans with PTSD. I don't want a repeat of interference from Congress on this issue."

Department of VA Affairs secretary: "But isn't it our job to support our vets?"

OMB director: Look what happened when we had to cave in on the real effects of Agent Orange used in Vietnam. Every time you turn around, medical research has established another form of cancer associated with Agent Orange. We cut off claims for that before we were forced to pay out billions to vets in compensation and benefits."

Department of VA Affairs secretary: "Are you telling me that because allowing compensation and benefits for PTSD, we are going to lose billions more?"

OMB director: "Of course! PTSD isn't even a physical injury! Go back and tell the assistant secretary for Veterans Benefits Administration and Healthcare Administration to deny those claims. The president wants budget money allocated to other projects."

Most directions of the OMB have behaved as if the government budget is their personal funds that should not be given away as if it was a public charity.

Another policy change that works against the veteran is not covered by the VA's self-congratulatory fact sheet. The Federal Circuit ruled in 2000 that denial of a claim is premature before the expiration of the one year period established by the Veterans Claims Assistance Act of 2000. However, the executive management level of the Department of Veterans Affairs lobbied Congress to insert a policy change in the Veterans Benefits Act of 2003 in which the VA can now deny a claim without waiting a full year. This is disturbing and unfair. Supposing you file a claim lacking certain evidence to support your argument. The VA adjudicator sends you a letter stating the evidence he requires and gives you a suspense date of sixty to ninety days to produce it. You are unsuccessful in obtaining this information within the time frame; thus, your claim goes into the automatic claim-denial mode.

How a PTSD Claim Is Decided

Now we want to take a look at the administrative side of the equation. In deciding the merits of a PTSD claim, the rating board member must apply five sets of guidelines to each claim he reviews: *U.S. Code Title 38*, sections 1110, 1131, 1154(b), 5103, 5103A, 5104, 5107, and 5109; *Code of Federal Regulations* volume 1, parts 3 and 4; VA Manual M21-1, part VI, subchapter 11, section 11.37, opinions provided by the Office of General Counsel (OGC), Department of Veterans Affairs; and rulings passed by the U.S. Court of Appeals for Veterans Claims (USCAVC).

In theory, if the guidelines in each of these sources are applied correctly, there should seldom be a need for someone to appeal a decision. As you read through statutes to the *CFRs*, the manuals, and the general council opinions, notice the changing interpretation of the guidelines.

But, in fairness, it is the veteran who makes it possible for claims examiners to turn down so many claims. The hit song, "You Gotta Know the Territory" from *The Music Man* is right on point. You have to know how to implement your rights. *Only you can do this.* If you say to them: "Hey! You didn't do this or that, which is why you mishandled my claim," the next time claims examiners review it, they will pay attention. No one likes to look like an idiot to those who sit on the thrones of upper management.

Title 38 U.S. Code: Veterans Benefits

Title 38 U.S. Code, "Veterans Benefits," is a codification of veterans' affairs laws that are under the jurisdiction of the Committee on Veterans' Affairs of the U.S. House of Representatives and the U.S. Senate. These statutes are the laws for providing compensation benefits. They are for all veterans who have, in one way or another, become disabled because of an in-service injury or illness.

SECTION 1131: BASIC ENTITLEMENT (LAST AMENDED IN 2003)
The full text of this section reads as follows:

> For disability resulting from personal injury suffered or disease contracted in line of duty, or for aggravation of a preexisting injury suffered or disease contracted in line of duty, in the active military, naval, or air service, during other than a period of war, the United States will pay to any veteran thus disabled and who was discharged or released under conditions other than dishonorable from the period of service in which said injury or disease was incurred, or preexisting

injury or disease was aggravated, compensation as provided in this subchapter, but no compensation shall be paid if the disability is a result of the veteran's own willful misconduct or abuse of alcohol or drugs.

SECTION 1154(B): CONSIDERATION TO BE ACCORDED TIME, PLACE, AND CIRCUMSTANCES OF SERVICE

The text of this section reads as follows:

> In the case of any *veteran who engaged in combat* with the enemy in active service with a military, naval, or air organization of the United States during a period of war, campaign, or expedition, *the Secretary shall accept as sufficient proof of service connection of any disease or injury alleged* to have been *incurred in or aggravated* by such service satisfactory lay or other evidence of service incurrence or aggravation of such injury or disease, *if consistent with the circumstances, conditions, or hardships of such service*, notwithstanding the fact that there is no official record of such incurrence or aggravation in such service, and, *to that end, shall resolve every reasonable doubt in favor of the veteran.* Service connection of such injury or disease may be rebutted by clear and convincing evidence to the contrary. The reasons for granting or denying service-connection in each case shall be recorded in full. (Italics added.)

The last time this particular statute was amended was August 6, 1991. Certain words in this passage have been italicized for emphasis. These are the words are needed to request further action when your claim is denied; that is, these words are your Bill of Rights. Know them so that if the VA steps out of line—by denying your legitimate claim—you can successfully defend your claim by showing how the VA guidelines were not followed.

SECTION 5103: NOTICE TO CLAIMANTS OF REQUIRED INFORMATION AND EVIDENCE (2004)

The text of this section reads as follows:

(a) Required information and evidence.
Upon receipt of a complete or substantially complete application, the Secretary shall notify the claimant and the claimant's representative, if any, of any information, and any medical or lay evidence, not previously provided to the Secretary that is necessary to substantiate the claim. As part of that notice, the Secretary shall indicate which portion of that information and evidence, if any, is to be provided by the claimant and which portion, if any, the Secretary, in accordance with section 5103A of this title and any other applicable provisions of law, will attempt to obtain on behalf of the claimant.

(b) Time limitation.

(1) In the case of information or evidence that the claimant is notified under subsection (a) is to be provided by the claimant, such information or evidence must be received by the Secretary within one year from the date such notice is sent.

(2) This subsection shall not apply to any application or claim for Government life insurance benefits.

(3) Nothing in paragraph (1) shall be construed to prohibit the Secretary from making a decision on a claim before the expiration of the period referred to in that subsection.

When the VA claims examiner writes for information or to establish a time requirement, you are expected to react before the expiration date unless you wish to invite a denial of benefits.

SECTION 5103A: DUTY TO ASSIST CLAIMANTS
Full text of this section reads as follows:

(a) Duty to assist.

(1) The Secretary shall make reasonable efforts to assist a claimant in obtaining evidence necessary to substantiate the claimant's claim for a benefit under a law administered by the Secretary.

(2) The Secretary is not required to provide assistance to a claimant under this section if no reasonable possibility exists that such assistance would aid in substantiating the claim.

(3) The Secretary may defer providing assistance under this section pending the submission by the claimant of essential information missing from the claimant's application.

(b) Assistance in obtaining records.

(1) As part of the assistance provided under subsection (a), the Secretary shall make reasonable efforts to obtain relevant records (including private records) that the claimant adequately identifies to the Secretary and authorizes the Secretary to obtain.

(2) Whenever the Secretary, after making such reasonable efforts, is unable to obtain all of the relevant records sought, the Secretary shall notify the claimant that the Secretary is unable to obtain records with respect to the claim. Such a notification shall

(A) identify the records the Secretary is unable to obtain;

(B) briefly explain the efforts that the Secretary made to obtain those records; and

(C) describe any further action to be taken by the Secretary with respect to the claim.

(3) Whenever the Secretary attempts to obtain records from a Federal department or agency under this subsection or subsection (c), the efforts to obtain those records shall continue until the records are obtained unless it is reasonably certain that such records do not exist or that further efforts to obtain those records would be futile.

(c) Obtaining records for compensation claims.
In the case of a claim for disability compensation, the assistance provided by the Secretary under subsection (b) shall include obtaining the following records if relevant to the claim:

(1) the claimants service medical records and, if the claimant has furnished the Secretary information sufficient to locate such records, other relevant records pertaining to the claimant's active military, naval, or air service that are held or maintained by a governmental entity;

(2) records of relevant medical treatment or examination of the claimant at Department healthcare faculties or at the expense of the Department, if the claimant furnishes information sufficient to locate those records;

(3) any other relevant records held by any Federal department or agency that the claimant adequately identifies and authorizes the Secretary to obtain.

(d) Medical examinations for compensation claims.

(1) In the case of a claim for disability compensation, the assistance provided by the Secretary under subsection (a) shall include providing a medical examination or obtaining a medical opinion when such an examination or opinion is necessary to make a decision on the claim.

(2) The Secretary shall treat an examination or opinion as being necessary to make a decision on a claim for purposes of paragraph (1) if the evidence of record before the Secretary, taking into consideration all information and lay or medical evidence (including statements of the claimant)

(A) contains competent evidence that the claimant has a current disability, or persistent or recurrent symptoms of disability; and

(B) indicates that the disability or symptoms may be associated with the claimant's active military, naval, or air service; but

(C) does not contain sufficient medical evidence for the Secretary to make a decision on the claim.

(e) Regulations.
The Secretary shall prescribe regulations to carry out this section.

(f) Rule with respect to disallowed claims.
Nothing in this section shall be construed to require the Secretary to reopen a claim that has been disallowed except when new and material evidence is presented or secured, as described in section 5108 of this title.

(g) Other assistance not precluded.
Nothing in this section shall be construed as precluding the Secretary from providing such other assistance under subsection (a) to a claimant in substantiating a claim as the Secretary considers appropriate.

SECTION 5104: DECISIONS AND NOTICES OF DECISIONS
Full text of this section reads as follows:

(a) In the case of a decision by the Secretary under section 511 of this title affecting the provision of benefits to a claimant, the Secretary shall, on a timely basis, provide to the claimant (and to the claimant's representative) notice of such decision. The notice shall include an explanation of the procedure for obtaining review of the decision.
(b) In any case where the Secretary denies a benefit sought, the notice required by subsection (a) shall also include:
    (1) a statement of the reasons for the decision, and
    (2) a summary of the evidence considered by the Secretary.

This is one of those rules you must be aware of. Any time the VA denies your claim without including the documents outlined in section (b) above, immediately file a Notice of Disagreement.

SECTION 5107: CLAIMANT RESPONSIBILITY; BENEFIT OF THE DOUBT
Full text of this section reads as follows:

(a) Claimant responsibility.
Except as otherwise provided by law, a claimant has the responsibility to present and support a claim for benefits under laws administered by the Secretary.

(b) Benefit of the doubt.
The Secretary shall consider all information and lay and medical evidence of record in a case before the Secretary with respect to benefits under laws administered by the Secretary. When there is an approximate balance of positive and negative evidence regarding any issue material to the determination of a matter, the Secretary shall give the benefit of the doubt to the claimant.

The benefit of doubt law says that before the VA can deny your claim it must prove that its evidence is superior to yours. The VA can't say it considered all the evidence and a preponderance is against your claim. It must say exactly what evidence it has and why this evidence is superior. Be warned: claims officers disregard this requirement on a regular basis.

SECTION 5109: INDEPENDENT MEDICAL OPINIONS
Full text of this section reads as follows:

(a) When, in the judgment of the Secretary, expert medical opinion, in addition to that available within the Department, is warranted by the medical complexity or controversy involved in a case being considered by the Department, the Secretary may secure an advisory medical opinion from one or more independent medical experts who are not employees of the Department.

(b) The Secretary shall make necessary arrangements with recognized medical schools, universities, or clinics to furnish such advisory medical opinions. Any such arrangement shall provide that the actual selection of the expert or experts to give the advisory opinion in an individual case shall be made by an appropriate official of such institution.

(c) The Secretary shall furnish a claimant with notice that an advisory medical opinion has been requested under this section with respect to the claimant's case and shall furnish the claimant with a copy of such opinion when it is received by the Secretary.

Treatment of veterans with PTSD is, at its very core, appalling. Why has the U.S. Court of Appeals for Veterans Claims revisited the issue of PTSD nearly 900 times? One reason is that diagnosing PTSD is not a black and white medical issue. Another reason is that both parties contribute to the confusion. The typical veteran has no idea what constitutes a valid claim. All he does know that he is a victim of PTSD, but for various reasons he is unable to speak about it to the outside world. On top of this, he is ill-prepared to cope with the administrative and technical realities of a giant bureaucracy. When he does reach out, he puts his trust in the VA to do the right thing.

Very few VA claims examiners have experienced a traumatic, life-threatening event that would give them some insight into the experiences of a veteran with PTSD. Remember my friend from chapter 3, Sgt. David Raz? He is a victim of VA bias. It appears that PTSD claims are rated by narrowest interpretation of the laws, regulations, and evidence.

What to Do If the VA Sends You a Rejection Letter

These points should be kept in mind if your claim for PTSD is denied:

◆   The RO's decisions must be based only on the evidence contained in the claim file. This is mandated by Title 38 U.S. Code.

◆   If the claimed stressor is not combat related, your statement alone is not sufficient to establish a well-grounded claim.

◆   There are three elements that must be proved to establish service connection for PTSD. (1) There must a current medical diagnosis that the PTSD is active. (2) The veteran must show the condition was the result of his military service. (3) A link between the current medical symptoms and the incident that caused the PTSD must be shown. A cook, for example, has to prove that he was shot at on guard duty and that that incident was the cause of his PTSD. A cook is not considered a combatant; therefore, he has to prove both that he is currently disabled by PTSD and that someone actually shot at him. The proof is the nexus that ties it all together.

◆   Rating boards and the BVA are required by law to account for all the evidence both persuasive and unpersuasive. It must give reasons for rejecting any evidence supporting the veteran's claim.

◆   Just because the RO cannot find evidence in the veteran's military service records (service medical records, or SMRs) does not exempt claims examiners from appraising the value of other evidence in determining service connection.

◆   All evidence is presumed to be true when a the board considers whether or not a claim is well grounded.

The VA must assist the veteran with his claim by obtaining records, advising what other evidence may be necessary, and scheduling him for a C&P examination. Do not expect more than a cursory search for records. In all the years I've been dealing with the VA, I never saw a case where claims examiners have requested morning reports, organization histories, after action reports, or military hospital records to help a veteran make a case for his claim.

38 Code of Federal Regulations

The next step in the administrative process is publishing a regulation that spells out in greater detail the intent of Congress. Congress will pass a specific "act" pertaining to one of the three branches of government. That new law is assigned to the appropriate government agency, and each department or agency is responsible for authoring a corresponding statute. The section pertinent to the Department of Veterans Affairs is known as *38 Code of Federal Regulations (38 CFR)* and is published annually. These regulations should make clear what Congress intended when it passed the initial act, and the individual department cannot add new language that totally disregards Congress's original meaning.

The pertinent regulations are provided in as follows.

38 *CFR* §3.304: DIRECT SERVICE CONNECTION; WARTIME AND PEACETIME (2003)

(c) Development.

The development of evidence in connection with claims for service connection will be accomplished when deemed necessary but *it should not be undertaken when evidence present is sufficient for this determination.* In initially rating disability of record at the time of discharge, the records of the service department, including the reports of examination at enlistment and the clinical records during service, will ordinarily suffice. Rating of combat injuries or other conditions which obviously had their inception in service may be accomplished pending receipt of copy of the examination at enlistment and all other service records.

(d) Combat.

Satisfactory lay or other evidence that an injury or disease was incurred or aggravated in combat will be accepted as sufficient proof of service connection if the evidence is consistent with the circumstances, conditions, or hardships of the veteran's service even though there is no official record of such incurrence.

(f) Post-traumatic stress disorder.

Service connection for post traumatic stress disorder requires medical evidence diagnosing the condition in accordance with Sec. 4.125(a) of this chapter; a link, established by medical evidence, between current symptoms and an in-service stressor; and credible supporting evidence that the claimed in-service stressor occurred. Although service connection may be established based on other in-service stressors, the following provisions apply for specified in-service stressors as set forth below:

(1) If the evidence establishes that the veteran engaged in combat with the enemy and the claimed stressor is related to that combat, in the absence of clear and convincing evidence to the contrary, and provided that the claimed stressor is consistent with the circumstances, conditions, or hardships of the veteran's service, the veteran's lay testimony alone may establish the occurrence of the claimed in-service stressor.

(2) If the evidence establishes that the veteran was a prisoner-of-war under the provisions of Sec. 3.1(y) of this part and the claimed stressor is related to that prisoner-of-war experience, in the absence of clear and convincing evidence to the contrary, and provided that the claimed stressor is consistent with the

circumstances, conditions, or hardships of the veteran's service, the veteran's lay testimony alone may establish the occurrence of the claimed in-service stressor.

38 *CFR* §3.326: EXAMINATIONS

For purposes of this section, the term examination includes periods of hospital observation when required by VA.

(a) Where there is a claim for disability compensation or pension but medical evidence accompanying the claim is not adequate for rating purposes, a Department of Veterans Affairs examination will be authorized. This paragraph applies to original and reopened claims as well as claims for increase submitted by a veteran, surviving spouse, parent, or child. Individuals for whom an examination has been scheduled are required to report for the examination.

(b) Provided that it is otherwise adequate for rating purposes, any hospital report, or any examination report, from any government or private institution may be accepted for rating a claim without further examination. However, monetary benefits to a former Prisoner of War will not be denied unless the claimant has been offered a complete physical examination conducted at a Department of Veterans Affairs hospital or outpatient clinic.

(c) Provided that it is otherwise adequate for rating purposes, a statement from a private physician may be accepted for rating a claim without further examination.

38 *CFR* §3.340: TOTAL AND PERMANENT RATINGS AND UNEMPLOYABILITY

(a) Total disability ratings.

(1) General. Total disability will be considered to exist when there is present any impairment of mind or body which is sufficient to render it impossible for the average person to follow a substantially gainful occupation. Total disability may or may not be permanent. Total ratings will not be assigned, generally, for temporary exacerbations or acute infectious diseases except where specifically prescribed by the schedule.

(2) Schedule for rating disabilities. Total ratings are authorized for any disability or combination of disabilities for which the Schedule for Rating Disabilities prescribes a 100% evaluation or, with less disability, where the requirements of paragraph 16, page 5 of the rating schedule are present or where, in pension cases, the requirements of paragraph 17, page 5 of the schedule are met.

(3) Ratings of total disability on history. In the case of disabilities which have undergone some recent improvement, a rating of total disability may be made, provided:

(i) That the disability must in the past have been of sufficient severity to warrant a total disability rating;

(ii) That it must have required extended, continuous, or intermittent hospitalization, or have produced total industrial incapacity for at least one year, or be subject to recurring, severe, frequent, or prolonged exacerbations; and

(iii) That it must be the opinion of the rating agency that despite the recent improvement of the physical condition, the veteran will be unable to effect an adjustment into a substantially gainful occupation. Due consideration will be given to the frequency and duration of totally incapacitating exacerbations since incurrence of the original disease or injury, and to periods of hospitalization for treatment in determining whether the average person could have reestablished himself or herself in a substantially gainful occupation.

(b) Permanent total disability.

Permanence of total disability will be taken to exist when such impairment is reasonably certain to continue throughout the life of the disabled person. The permanent loss or loss of use of both hands, or of both feet, or of one hand and one foot, or of the sight of both eyes, or becoming permanently helpless or bedridden constitutes permanent total disability. Diseases and injuries of long standing which are actually totally incapacitating will be regarded as permanently and totally disabling when the probability of permanent improvement under treatment is remote. Permanent total disability ratings may not be granted as a result of any incapacity from acute infectious disease, accident, or injury, unless there is present one of the recognized combinations or permanent loss of use of extremities or sight, or the person is in the strict sense permanently helpless or bedridden, or when it is reasonably certain that a subsidence of the acute or temporary symptoms will be followed by irreducible totality of disability by way of residuals. The age of the disabled person may be considered in determining permanence.

(c) Insurance ratings.

A rating of permanent and total disability for insurance purposes will have no effect on ratings for compensation or pension.

[26 FR 1585, Feb. 24, 1961, as amended at 46 FR 47541, Sept. 29, 1981]

38 *CFR* §4.18: UNEMPLOYABILITY

A veteran may be considered as unemployable upon termination of employment which was provided on account of disability or in which special consideration was given on account of the same when it is satisfactorily shown that he or she is unable to secure further employment. With amputations, sequelae of fractures, and other residuals of traumatism shown to be of static character, a showing of continuous Unemployability from date of incurrence, or the date the condition reached the stabilized level, is a general requirement in order to establish the fact that present unemployability is the result of the disability. However, consideration is to be given to the circumstances of employment in individual claims, and, if the employment was only occasional, intermittent, tryout or unsuccessful, or eventually terminated on account of the disability, present unemployability may be attributed to the static disability. Where unemployability for pension previously has been established on the basis of combined service-connected and non-service-connected disabilities and the service-connected disability or disabilities have increased in severity, Sec. 4.16 is for consideration.

[40 FR 42536, Sept. 15, 1975, as amended at 43 FR 45349, Oct. 2, 1978]

38 *CFR* §4.125: DIAGNOSIS OF MENTAL DISORDERS

(a) If the diagnosis of a mental disorder does not conform to DSM-IV or is not supported by the findings on the examination report, the rating agency shall return the report to the examiner to substantiate the diagnosis.

(b) If the diagnosis of a mental disorder is changed, the rating agency shall determine whether the new diagnosis represents progression of the prior diagnosis, correction of an error in the prior diagnosis, or development of a new and separate condition. If it is not clear from the available records what the change of diagnosis represents, the rating agency shall return the report to the examiner for a determination.

(Authority: 38 U.S.C. 1155)

[61 FR 52700, Oct. 8, 1996]

Regulations are specific laws that are turned into working legal instructions. These regulations have the power of law for the agency, employees, and veterans. When two people (e.g., the VA claims examiners and a veteran) have a different conception of what the regulation dictates, the Board of Veterans or the U.S. Court of Appeals for Veterans Claims resolves the issue.

VA Manual M21-1

Subchapter 11, paragraph 11.37 answers the rater's question: "What am I suppose to do when rating PTSD claims?" After you read some case summaries of the U.S. Court of Appeals for Veterans Claims in chapter 12, you have to wonder how they arrive at some of the decisions they publish. Here is the full text from VA Manual M21-1, part III, chapter 5, paragraph 5.14 and part VI, chapter 11, paragraph 11.37 (directly quoted or, in places, amended for clarity).

5.14 POST-TRAUMATIC STRESS DISORDER

Post-traumatic stress disorder. Service connection for post-traumatic stress disorder (PTSD) requires medical evidence diagnosing the condition in accordance with 38 *CFR* 4.125(a), a link, established by medical evidence, between current symptoms and an in-service stressor, and credible evidence that the claimed in-service stressor occurred (38 *CFR* 3 304(f)).

Evidence of a stressor in service. Obtain all available evidence from the service department showing that the veteran served "where the stressful event occurred. Also obtain evidence supporting the veteran's description of the event.

(1) Combat Stressors. The following individual decorations are examples of decorations which may serve as evidence that the veteran engaged in combat:

- Air Force Cross
- Air Medal with "V" Device
- Army Commendation Medal with "V" Device
- Bronze Star- Medal with "V" Device
- Combat Action Ribbon
- Combat Infantryman Badge
- Combat Medical Badge
- Distinguished Flying Cross
- Distinguished Service Cross
- Joint Service Commendation Medal with "V" Device
- Medal of Honor
- Navy Commendation Medal with "V" Device
- Navy Cross
- Purple Heart
- Silver Star.

If the evidence established that the veteran engaged in combat with the enemy and the claimed stressor is related to that combat, in the absence of clear and convincing evidence to the contrary—and provided that the claimed stressor is consistent with the circumstances, conditions, or hardships of the veteran's service—the veteran's testimony alone establishes the occurrences of the claimed in-service stressor. (38 *CFR* 3.30 4(f) and 38 USC 1154(b)).

(2) Noncombat Stressors. PTSD may result from a noncombat stressor, such as: a plane crash, ship sinking, explosion, rape or assault, duty on a burn ward or in a graves registration unit.

(3) POW Status. If the evidence establishes that the veteran was a Prisoner of War under the provisions if 38 *CFR*3.1(y) and the claimed stressor is related to that [POW] experience, in the absence of clear and convincing evidence to the contrary and provided that the claimed stressor is consistent with the circumstances conditions or hardships of the veteran's service, the veteran's testimony alone establishes the occurrence of the claimed in-service stressor, 3M *CFR* 3.304(f) and 38 U.S.C 1154(b).

Development.

(1) If the veteran indicates pertinent treatment in a VA facility, Vet Center, or elsewhere, request hospital report(s) and clinical records.

(2) If the evidence does not establish that the veteran was engaged in combat with the enemy, or the evidence does establish this but the claimed stressor is not related to that combat, then credible supporting evidence is required to establish that a stressor occurred, 38 *CFR* 3.304(f). In cases where available records do not contain this develop for this evidence as follows:

(a) Request specific details of the in-service stressful incident(s) date(s), places(s), unit of assignment at the time of the event(s), description of the event(s), medal(s) or citation(s) received as a result of the event(s) and if appropriate name other identifying information concerning other individuals involved in the event(s). As a minimum, the claim must indicate the location and approximate time (a 2-month specific date range) of the stressful event(s) in question, and the unit of assignment at he time the stressful event occurred. Inform the veteran that this information is necessary to obtain supportive evidence of the stressful event(s) and that failure to respond or an incomplete response may result in denial of the claim.

Note: Do not ask the veteran for specific details in any case in which there is credible supporting evidence that the claimed in-service stressor occurred.

(b) Use only the codes at the time in PIES. Use O19 for simple PTSD claims and 018 for personal trauma. Do *not* use free text and list all of the information mentioned in the in manual. The response team at NPRC knows which pages to send for simple PTSI cases. In personal trauma cases, they will send copies of everything. There should be no occasion where both 018 and 019 are used. *If the claim is for both personal trauma and PTSD, the use of code 018 will include pages that would have sent in response to code 019. In either event, no additional* instructions need to be added to the PIES request. (Italics added.)

♦ **ARMY:** Personnel Qualification Record DA Form 2-1. The form is used for both Officers and Enlisted personnel and first came into use in January 1973. Prior to that DA Form 20 and DA Form 66 were used.

- **NAVY:** Enlisted record of "Transfer and Receipts (pp. 1, 32– 33). Enlisted record of "Administrative Remarks" (pp. 4–9, 34) Officer record, NAVPERS 1301/51. "Officer Data Card," (p. 35). DD 214 and enlistment contracts are usually included.
- **AIR FORCE:** "Airman Military Record," AF Form 7, Enlisted (pp. 36 –39); AF Form 11, Officer (pp. 39–40). Performance reports are for both Officer and Enlisted.
- **MARINE CORPS:** Enlistment contracts discharge Papers, MABMC-11 (discharge order) and service records are usually provided (pp. 3, 5–6, 8–9, 12–13, 17).
- **COAST GUARD:** Enlisted Record, "Endorsement on Order Sheet" (DOT Form GC 3312B). Officer Record, "Service Records Card, CG 3301, CG 3313, and CG 3305 (pp. 3, 5, 6–7), DD-214 and enlistment contract.

(3) If medical evidence establishes a valid diagnosis of PTSD and development is complete in every respect but for confirmation of the service stressor, contact either the U.S. Armed Center for Unit Records Research (CURR or lay marine corps (subparagraph (3) (b) Requests to that office must include the following:

- a two-month specific date range when the stressful event occurred
- the veteran's unit of assignment at the time of the stressful event, and
- the geographic location where the stressful event took place.

Additional information identified by CURR as helpful in conducting research includes:

- medals or citations received by the veteran; and
- stressful events witnessed by the veteran. Specific information including the names of other soldiers or sailors' involved, dates, units of assignment, and their geographic location is essential.

Note: CURR maintains a database of pending research requests. Any research requests identified as inadequate will be closed out. Additional development should be undertaken prior resubmission of the request to CURR. Stations may, at their discretion, render a final decision on cases if they determine that the information needed to conduct research is unobtainable. The file should be documented to this effect.

(a) For all services except the marine corps send the letter to: U.S. Armed Services Center for Unit Records Research (CURR), 7798 Cissna Road, Suite 101, Springfield, VA, 221511-3197. Telephone numbers are 703-806-7835 or 703-806-7838. If necessary, you may also contact the Coast Guard at Commander,

Military Personnel Command. MPC–S3, 2100 (H) Second St. SW, Washington, DC, 20593-0001.

(b) For U.S. Marine Corps veterans with service after 1956, send the letter to: Commandant of the Marine Corps Headquarters U.S. Marine Corps MMSB10, 2008 Elliot Road, Suite 201, Quantico, VA 22134-5030. Telephone numbers are 703-784-3935, 703-784-3935, or 703-784-3940. For veterans with service before 1956, send to: Marine Corps Historical Center, Building 58, Washington Navy Yard, Washington, DC, 20374-9580. Telephone number is 202-433-3840. All command chronologies are located at the Historical Center as well as unit diaries before 1956 and some unit diaries for the period 1956 to 1966. Quantico should have all unit diaries from 1956 on. In some instances, the military may forward the RO's inquiry to the other facility for a better answer.

(c) Enclose copies of information received from the veteran and the service department with these requests. These letters should *not* be sent until a *valid* diagnosis of PTSD is of record.

(4) If sufficient evidence is already of record to grant service connection for a claimed condition, do so. If not, but there is a continued diagnosis of PTSD, send an inquiry to the CURR or the marine corps. However, always send an inquiry for instances in which the only obstacle to service connection is confirmation of an alleged stressor. A denial solely because of an unconfirmed stressor is improper unless it has first been reviewed by the CURR or the marine corps.

(5) Occasionally the CURR or the marine corps will request a more specific description of the stressor in question. Failure of the veteran to respond substantively to the request for information will be grounds to deny the claim based on unconfirmed stressors.

PTSD claims based on personal assault.

(1) Veterans claiming service connection for disability owing to an in-service personal assault face unique problems in documenting their claims. Personal assault is an event of human design that threatens or inflicts harm. Examples of this are rape, physical assault, domestic battering, robbery, mugging, and stalking. Although these incidents are most often thought of as involving female veterans, male veterans can also be involved. Care must be taken to tailor development for a male or female veteran. These incidents are often violent and may lead to the development of PTSD secondary to personal assault.

(2) Because assault is an extremely personal and sensitive issue, many incidents of personal assault are not officially reported, and victims of this type of

in-service trauma may find it difficult to produce evidence to support the occurrence of the stressor. Therefore, alternative evidence must be sought.

(3) To service connect PTSD there must be credible evidence to support the veteran's assertion that the stressful event occurred. This does not mean that the evidence actually proves that the incident occurred; rather there should be at least an approximate balance of positive and negative evidence that it occurred.

(4) Review the claim and all its attached documents. Develop for SMRs and MPRJ information as needed.

(a) Service records not normally requested but may be needed to develop this type of claim. Responses to the development letter may identify additional information sources. These include:

- a rape crisis center or center for domestic abuse
- a counseling facility
- a health clinic
- family members or roommates
- a faculty member
- medical reports, civilian physicians or caregiver's who may have treated the veteran either immediately following the incident or sometime later
- a chaplain or clergy
- fellow service persons, or
- personal diaries or journals.

(b) Obtain any reports from military police, shore patrol, provost marshals office, or other military law enforcement. Development may include phone, fax, e-mail, or correspondence as long as they are documented in the file.

(5) Identifying possible sources of alternative evidence will require that you ask the veteran for information concerning the incident. This should he done as compassionately as possible in order to avoid further traumatization for PTSD stressor development letter used by regional offices to solicit details concerning a combat stressful incident is inappropriate for this type of PTSD claim. See a letter developed locally for this type of claim.

(6) Same development letters are inappropriate for PTSD claims based on personal assault and should not be used for that purpose. Instead use a letter or an attachment developed locally.

(7) Rating Veterans Service Representatives (RVSRS) must carefully evaluate all the available evidence. If the military record contains no documentation

that a personal assault occurred, alternate evidence might still establish an in-service stressful incident. Behavior changes that occurred at the time of the incident may indicate the occurrence of an in-service stressor. Examples of behavior changes that might indicate a stressor are but not limited to:

(a) visits to a medical or counseling clinic or dispensary without a specific diagnosis or specific ailment;

(b) sudden requests that the veteran's military occupational series or duty assignment be changed without other justification;

(c) lay statements indicating increased use or abuse of leave without an apparent reason such as family obligations or family illness;

(d) changes in performance and performance evaluations;

(e) lay statements describing episodes of depression, panic attacks, or anxiety but with no identifiable reasons for the episodes;

(f) increased or decreased use of prescription medications;

(g) increased use of over-the-counter medications;

(h) evidence of' substances abuse such as alcohol or drugs;

(i) increased disregard for military or civilian authority;

(j) obsessive behavior such as overeating or under-eating;

(k) pregnancy tests around the time of the incident;

(l) increased interest in tests for HIV or sexually transmitted diseases;

(m) unexplained economic or social behavior changes;

(n) treatment for physical injuries around the time of the veteran's claimed trauma but not reported as a result of the trauma; and

(o) breakup of a primary relationship.

(8) In personal assault claims, secondary evidence may need interpretation by a specialist if it involves behavior changes. Evidence that documents such behavior changes may require interpretation in relationship to the medical diagnosis by a neuropsychiatric physician.

11.37 POST-TRAUMATIC STRESS DISORDER (PTSD)

Service connection for PTSD requires medical evidence establishing a clear diagnosis of the condition, credible supporting evidence that the claimed in-service stressor actually occurred, and a link (established by medical evidence) between current symptomatology and the claimed in-service stressor (38 *CFR* 3.304(f)). The issue of service connection for PTSD is the sole responsibility of the rating specialist at the local level. Central Office opinion or guidance may be requested on complex cases.

Stressors.

In making a decision, exercise fair, impartial, and reasonable judgment in determining whether a specific case of PTSD is service connected. Some relevant considerations are:

(1) PTSD does not need to have its onset during combat. For example, vehicular or airplane crashes, large fires, flood, earthquakes, and other disasters evoke significant distress in most involved persons. The trauma may be experienced alone (rape or assault) or in the company of groups of people (military combat).

(2) A stressor is not to be limited to a single episode. A group of experiences also may affect an individual, leading to a diagnosis of PTSD in some circumstances—for example, assignment to a grave registration unit, burn cam unit, or liberation of internment camps could have a cumulative effect of powerful, distressing experiences essential to a diagnosis of PTSD.

(3) PTSD can be caused by events that occurred before, during, or after service. The relationship between stressors during military service and current problems/symptoms will govern the question of service connection. Symptoms must have a clear relationship to the military stressor as described in the medical reports.

(4) PTSD can occur hours, months, or years after a military stressor. Despite this long latent period, service-connected PTSD may be recognizable by a relevant association between the stressor and the current presentation of symptoms. This association between stressor and symptoms must be specifically addressed in the VA examination report and to a practical extent supported by documentation.

(5) Every decision involving the issue of service connection for PTSD alleged to have occurred as a result of combat must include a factual determination as to whether or not a veteran was engaged in combat, including the reasons or bases for that finding (see *Gaines v. West, 111 Vet. App. 113, 1998*).

Evidence of stressors in service.

(1) Conclusive Evidence. Any evidence available from the service department indicating that the veteran served in the area in which the stressful event is alleged to have occurred and any evidence supporting the description of the event are to be made part of the record. Corroborating evidence of a stressor is not restricted to service records, but *may* be obtained from other sources (see *Doran v. Brown, 6 Vet. App. 283, (1994)*. If the claimed stressor is related to combat, in the absence of information to the contrary, receipt of any of the following individual decorations will be considered evidence that a veteran engaged in combat:

- ◆ Air Force Cross
- ◆ Air Medal with "V" Device
- ◆ Army Commendation Medal with "V" Device

- Bronze Star Medal with "V" Device
- Combat Action Ribbon
- Combat Infantryman Badge
- Combat Medical Badge
- Combat Aircrew Insignia
- Distinguished Flying Cross
- Distinguished Service Cross
- Joint Service Commendation Medal with "V" Device
- Medal of Honor
- Navy Commendation Medal with "V" Device
- Navy Cross
- Purple Heart
- Silver Star.

Other supportive evidence includes but is not limited to plane crash, ship sinking, explosion, rape or assault, duty on a burn ward or in graves registration unit, POW status that satisfies the requirements of 38 *CFR* 3.1(y). These will also be considered conclusive evidence of an in-service stressor.

(2) Evidence of Personal Assault. Personal assault is an event of human design that threatens or inflicts harm. Examples of this are rape, physical assault, domestic battering, robbery, mugging, and stalking.

(a) Alternative Evidence. If the military record contains no documentation that a personal assault occurred, alternative evidence might still establish an in-service stressful incident. Examples of such evidence include but are not limited to:

- records from law enforcement authorities;
- records from rape crisis centers, hospitals, or physicians;
- pregnancy tests or tests for sexually transmitted diseases; and
- statements from family members, roommates, fellow service members or clergy.

(b) Behavior Changes. Behavior changes that occurred at the time of the incident may indicate the occurrence of an in-service stressor. Examples of such changes include but are not limited to:

- visits to a medical or counseling clinic or dispensary without a specific diagnosis or specific ailment;
- sudden requests for a change in occupational series or duty assignment without other justification;
- increased use or abuse of leave without an apparent reason, such as family obligations or family illness;

- changes in performance and performance evaluations;
- episodes of depression, panic attacks, or anxiety but no identifiable reasons for the episodes;
- increased or decreased use of prescription medication;
- increased use of over-the-counter medications;
- substance abuse such as alcohol or drugs;
- increased disregard for military or civilian authority;
- obsessive behavior such as overeating or under-eating;
- unexplained economic or social behavior changes; and
- breakup of a primary relationship.

(c) Development Requirements. It is unlawful to deny a post-traumatic stress disorder claim that is based on in-service personal assault without first advising the claimant that evidence from sources other than service medical records, including evidence of behavior changes, may constitute credible supporting evidence of the stressor. The veteran should have the opportunity to furnish this type of evidence or indicate its potential sources.

(d) Interpretation of Secondary Evidence. In personal assault claims, secondary evidence may need interpretation by a clinician, especially if it involves behavior changes. Evidence that documents such behavior changes may require interpretation in relationship to the medical diagnosis or an opinion by an appropriate medical or mental health professional as to whether it indicates that a personal assault occurred.

(3) Credible Supporting Evidence. A combat veteran's lay testimony alone may establish an in-service stressor for purposes of service connecting PTSD *(Cohen* v. *Brown,* 94-661, U.S. Ct. Vet. App. March 7, 1997). However, a non-combat veteran's testimony alone does not qualify as "credible supporting evidence of the occurrence of an in-service stressor as required by *38 CFR 3.304(f)* After-the-fact psychiatric analyses that infer a traumatic event are likewise insufficient in this regard *(Moreau* v. *Brown, 9 Vet. App. 389, 1996).*

Development.
(1) For instructions regarding development of service records, medical treatment, and evidence of stressor or personal assault, refer to Part III, subparagraphs 5.14b and 5.14c.
(2) Unless medical evidence adequate for rating purposes is already of record, an immediate examination is needed. When requesting an examination, state in the remarks section of VA Form 21-2507, "Request for Physical Examination," "Claims folder to be made available to examiner upon request."

Incomplete examinations and/or reconciliation of diagnosis.
If an examination is received with the diagnosis of PTSI) that does not contain the above essentials of diagnosis, the claims examiner should return the examination as incomplete for rating purposes, note the deficiencies, and request reexamination.

(1) Examples of an unacceptable diagnosis include not only insufficient symptomatology but failure to identify or to adequately describe the stressor, or failure to consider prior reports demonstrating a mental disorder that could not support a diagnosis of PTSD. Conflicting diagnoses of record must be acknowledged and reconciled (by the claims examiner).

(2) The reviewer of claims should exercise caution to accurately define situational disturbances containing adjustment reaction of adult life, which subside when the situational disturbance no longer exists or is withdrawn, as well as the reactions of those without neurosis who have "dropped out" and have become alienated but are not afflicted with PTSD.

Link between in-service stressor and diagnosis.
Relevant specific information concerning what happened must be described along with as much detailed information as the veteran can provide to the examiner regarding time of the event (year, month, day), geographical location (corps, province, town, or other landmark feature such as a river or mountain), and the names of others who may have been involved in the incident. The examining psychiatrist or psychologist should comment on the presence or absence of other traumatic events and their relevance to the current symptoms. Service connection for PTSD will not be established either on the basis of a diagnosis of PTSD) unsupported by the type of history and description or where the examination and supporting material fill to indicate a link between current symptoms and an in-service stressful event(s).

Review of evidence.
(1) If a VA medical examination fails to establish a diagnosis of PTSD, the claim will be immediately denied on that basis. If no determination regarding the existence of a stressor has been made, a discussion of the alleged stressor need not be included in the rating decision.

(2) If the claimant has failed to provide a minimal description of the stressor (i.e., no indication of the time or place of a stressful event), the claim may be denied on that basis. The rating should specify the previous request for information.

(3) If a VA examination or other medical evidence establishes a valid diagnosis of PTSD, and development is complete in every respect but for confirmation

of the in-service stressor, additional evidence will be requested from either the Center for Unit Records Research (CURR) or marine corps. (See part III, paragraph 5.14.)

(4) A claims examiner should not send a case to the CURR or marine corps unless there is a confirmed diagnosis of PTSD adequate to establish entitlement to service connection. Correspondingly, an inquiry should always be sent in instances in which the only obstacle to service connection is confirmation of an alleged stressor. A denial by the claims examiner solely because of an unconfirmed stressor is improper unless it has first been reviewed by the CURR or marine corps.

(5) If the CURR or the marine corps requests a more specific description of the stressor in question, the veteran should immediately provide the necessary information. If the veteran provides a reasonably responsive reply, the claims examiner should forward it to the requesting agency. Failure by the veteran to respond substantively to the request for information will be grounds to deny the claim based on unconfirmed stressor. (See Part III, paragraph 5.14.)

When the VA denies a claim, it often makes mistakes in administrative procedures or in interpreting the intent of the law. VA manuals are big books of SOPs (Standard Operating Procedures) that spell out the ABCs of the regulations. The purpose of VA manuals is to provide the adjudication teams with detailed instructions about how they are to do their job. Knowing about the manuals' contents may be the difference between victory or defeat for a veteran.

Chapter 4: What Have We Learned?

1. "You've got to know the territory." This chapter is a map of the workings of the VA's adjudication process. *You can't defend what you don't know.* One reason why so many claims are denied or rated below their actual level of disability is because the claimant has no idea what the process is all about. You may think it's no fun reading all the pertinent laws, regulations, and manuals that apply to your claim. You're right! It doesn't beat a night on the town, but if you expect to receive your full benefits, you have to do it.

2. There are five primary groups of principle standards that govern the way the VA executes its duty to veterans. They are: statutes, regulations, manuals, general counsel opinions, and case law (see chapter 12). Failure of the VA claims examiners to properly execute the guidelines in any one of these regulatory standards is grounds for an appeal.

3. The VA has a duty to advise you of what information is required to support your claim. However, the process does not require providing details of how

you can find this information. VA Manual M21-1, part III, chapter 5, paragraph 5.14(c) spells out just what type of information is required and where to find it in the archives of the U.S. Government.

4. This is very important: When filing a PTSD claim, there are two steps you must follow: 1. Always file an informal claim first, as this gives you one year to accumulate all the evidence and protects your entitlement date. 2. Submit everything through your Senator or Congressional Representative. The VA response is much faster and they are less likely to dismiss your evidence when they know your claim is being followed by your legislator. The details of this procedure are discussed in chapter 10.

5. If you have been awarded any one of the medals listed in VA Manual 21-1, part III, chapter 5, paragraph 5.14(b)(1), your claim should be processed without making you prove your combat experiences. If you received a Bronze Star or Air Medal without a "V" Device, challenge the claims examiners if they don't accept this combat award as a combat stressor. Ask them what their legal authority is to exclude you from direct service connection when the Department of the Army awards the medal for meritorious service against the enemy. The bottom line is: in asking you to prove your combat experiences, they deliberately ignored a portion of 32 *CFR* §578.11 and §578.12.

6. When you are filing a claim for PTSD, it is absolutely essential that you are able to prove two important points. First, you must be currently diagnosed with PTSD; and, two, PTSD must be able to be traced back to your combat experiences.

7. Your chances of being awarded compensation benefits for PTSD improve considerably when a private sector psychiatrist evaluates you first. The purpose for this step is to take the initiative with the VA instead of waiting for a claims examiner to question your proof. Submitting a medical evaluation diagnosing PTSD with your claim application forces them to prove, by a preponderance of evidence, that this isn't true.

8. If you were previously denied compensation for PTSD, you might be able to reopen your claim because examiners failed to follow the court's decision in *Doran v. Brown*.[1] This case is discussed detail in chapter 12.

9. If the VA evaluation is conducted by anyone other than a psychiatrist or psychologist and the claim is denied, immediately notify the VA that you're appealing the decision because you were evaluated by a nonphysician. Remember, always ask the examiner what his or her medical credentials are. I once worked a case where they used a student resident from the local medical school to give a C&P examination.

Here is a list of the most common reasons VA adjudicators use when denying a PTSD claim:

- The declared stressor was not deemed as a possible cause of PTSD;
- Rating boards would not accept a diagnosis of PTSD as being substantiated;
- Rating boards would not accept alcoholism and drug addiction as a secondary condition to PTSD;
- Evidence, written or oral, given by the veteran was not given the proper weight and thus was not considered in the decision process;
- Evidence in the form of lay "buddy letters" was not accepted as evidence;
- Medical diagnosis and assessment by the veteran's own doctors were not accepted by rating board members;
- More often than not, rating boards held that other mental disorders were the cause of the veteran's conditions without considering the possibility that there could be multiple disorders for part of the veteran's illness;
- In many instances, rating board members would not assist in developing evidence related to the stressor once the veteran presented a well-grounded claim; rating board members would accept from VA C&P examiners reports that were not in compliance with their manuals and regulations.

Notes

1. *Doran v. Brown*, 6 F. 283 (Vet. App. 1994).

History of the Veterans Administration

The U.S veterans' benefits system traces its roots back to the seventeenth century when the pilgrims of Plymouth passed a law protecting citizens who joined the colony army to defend it against the hostile Pequot Indians. The colony ensured that any soldier disabled in its defense would be supported by the colony.

When the colonies united and declared their independence from England, the Continental Congress of 1776 also addressed the needs of its soldiers. To encourage enlistments during the Revolutionary War, Congress passed legislation authorizing pension benefits for soldiers. This was the first move by a fledgling republic to protect all citizens who took up arms to defend the republic.

Individual states and communities assumed responsibility for medical and hospital care for veterans in the early days of the republic. In 1811, the federal government authorized the first domiciliary and medical facility for veterans. Throughout the 1800s the nation's veterans assistance program expanded to include benefits and pensions not only for veterans, but also for their widows and dependents.

Following the Civil War, many states established homes for their veterans. Medical and hospital treatment was provided for all injuries and diseases, whether or not of service origin. Such homes cared for all homeless and disabled veterans of the Civil War, Indian Wars, Spanish-American War, and Mexican Border period, as well as those discharged from peacetime service.

When the United States entered World War I in 1917, Congress established a new system of veteran benefits. Programs included disability compensation, insurance for military members and vocational rehabilitation for the disabled. The swelling ranks of veterans in the 1920s led to the administration of benefits by three different federal agencies: the Veterans Bureau, the Bureau of Pensions of the Interior Department, and the National Home for Disabled Volunteer Soldiers. Yet veterans had to fend for themselves with each agency, each with its own laws and regulations. Many veterans wandered from agency to agency because of confusion and contradiction within the agencies about who was in charge.

In 1930, Congress authorized the president to consolidate and coordinate government activities affecting war veterans. The newly formed organization was known as the Veterans Administration. The three former agencies that independently exercised control over veteran's benefits were reassigned to the Veterans Administration and became bureaus within the new organization.

The Department of Veterans Affairs was established as a cabinet-level position on March 15, 1989. President George H. W. Bush hailed the creation of the new department saying, "There is only one place for the veterans of America, in the Cabinet Room, at the table with the President of the United States of America."[1] The first secretary of the Department of Veterans Affairs was former Republican Congressman Edward Joseph Derwinski. Despite President Bush's statement regarding the recognition of the VA, as of yet nothing of momentous proportion has escaped from the president's cabinet room to benefit veterans at large.

Despite the rhetoric of "We can't do enough for you," that has bombarded veterans since the early 1980s, benefits have been consistently downsized. Those ruling the executive branch since President Ronald Reagan have measured veterans' benefits only by bottom-line costs. Gone are the sincerity and pledges of a grateful nation for the sacrifices of those who have served. When politicians look at the fact that nearly twenty-seven million people have served in the military—in theory each has a potential claim for benefits—they see an immediate threat to their special interest projects.

At one time, it would have appeared un-American for any politician to announce benefits cuts for veterans. One might as well attack motherhood, apple pie, or the American flag. That was until President George W. Bush proclaimed in 2005 that domestic programs would have to take some heavy hits. The Office of Management and Budget is taking aim at veteran, social security, and education programs to offset the cost of the Iraq War, War on Terrorism, and continued tax cuts, while the national debt continues to grow larger.

The story in chapter 3 about Sgt. David Raz illustrates a covert way of cutting veterans benefits. Another measure, discussed in chapter 1, is to give different meanings to laws and regulations. The VA drags claims on endlessly before reaching a decision and hires rank and file of processing personnel with low-level technical skills. There has also been an effort to make VA compensation benefits taxable, which, if voted into law, would reduce the spendable income of the disabled. Some veterans must pay for their medication from the VA if the prescription is not directly linked to a service-connected condition. Veterans treated for illness or disease not designated service connected, and whose income is greater than the poverty level, must pay for their own care. If they have a private insurance company, their care could be charged against their policy. Because the VA cannot compete for highly skilled physicians, they hire foreign doctors, some with inadequate English-language skills, who will work for less than the going rate normally earned by physicians. The VA will accept language limitations in an effort to maintain hospital staffing requirements. They are also staffing VA medical positions with physician's assistants and nurse practitioners.

In order to cut costs, the VA has reduced the size and configuration of rating boards; doctors and lawyers are no longer members of the board, and now a single individual decides just about every type of claim considered by the former three-member board. Very few, if any, have the ability to evaluate complex medical issues requiring specialized training and experience.

The only event in 1989 that was truly helpful for veterans was the establishment of the U.S. Court of Appeals for Veterans Claims. No longer could the VA act as its own judge and jury in reviewing veterans' claims and benefits. The new federal court's only purpose was to ensure the laws and regulations pertaining to veterans' benefits were properly and fairly administered. The court has successfully reshaped the review process by the Board of Veterans' Appeals. The BVA is reversing and remanding appeals from Regional Offices (ROs) nationwide at an astounding rate.

Only a small percentage of veterans (20%) ever exercise their right of appeal.[2] *If every veteran who was turned down appealed the denial of benefits, the VA would buckle under the volume of appeals.* VA regional offices continue to ignore the decisions of the court; they fail to follow the regulations and laws and they do not decide claims based on precedent-setting case law, as mandated by the court. If the St. Petersburg RO followed the regulations and case law, Sgt. David Raz would not be passing his fifth year pursuing his benefits for PTSD.

Before filing any type of claim action with the VA, there are several fundamental concepts you need to know. Jesse Brown, former secretary of Department of Veterans Affairs, claims that the VA is user friendly. According to the *American Legion Magazine* (1995), "He does not believe that the Veterans Benefits Administration was systematically ignoring the law or the court."[3] He did not say, "I know they are *not* ignoring the law or the courts." For this reason, you and only you must take the time to understand how the VA operates, what its responsibilities are, and what proof you need for your claim. There are no shortcuts when it comes time to file a claim for your VA benefits.

Nine Types of Claim Actions

A veteran can file many types of claim actions with the VA. This book focuses on the four most important service-connected claim actions filed by a veteran. *It is absolutely necessary* that you know exactly what is entailed for the benefit you are claiming. Before you submit your claim, you must know what the law requires for that category of claim, as each category has special development techniques. One of the most basic and frequent mistakes made is requesting that a claim be "reopened" when the veteran actually wants to "amend" the claim. You must know what you want to claim and what the VA's responsibility is in responding to your request.

The nine categories of claims are:

- informal claim
- compensation claim
- claim for an increased rating
- reopened claim
- adjunct or secondary disabilities to original service-connected disability claim
- 100% total disability due to individual unemployability claim
- service connection for conditions resulting from medical treatment at VA hospital or clinics claim
- survivor's dependency and indemnity compensation claim
- nonservice-connected pension claims.

INFORMAL CLAIM: AN ANTI-DENIAL WEAPON

Anytime you are planning to file a claim, you should first file an *informal claim*. An informal claim establishes the claim entitlement date while you do the work of obtaining evidence and necessary documents. An informal claim is no more than a notice of intent to file a claim for benefits. It is simply a written notice such as:

> Please accept this notice as my informal claim for compensation benefits owing to a back injury I had while on active duty in 1967. I was treated for this condition at the VA hospital in Lake City, Florida, in 1968, Houston, Texas, in 1973, and the Bronx, New York, in 1980. A formal application will be filed once I have collected all of the evidence to support my claim for disability benefits.

This notice can be submitted on VA form 21-4138 "Statement in Support of Claim" or in a personal letter to the regional office.

ORIGINAL CLAIM

By definition, an original claim is the first claim filed for a particular benefit. Claims in this group must be first-time claims for service connection for a particular disease or injury as distinguished from a subsequent claim to reopen. An amendment to Title 38 U.S. Code declares that the VA has a statutory duty to assist you in the development of facts pertinent to your claim. This claim must be filed on VA form 21-521.

CLAIM FOR INCREASED BENEFITS

A claim for increased benefits is one of the most dangerous claim actions a veteran can file. If you think that your service-connected medical condition has increased in its severity, you may decide to file a claim for increased benefits. A majority of veterans base this decision on what they perceive as a deterioration of their health problem rather than on a current medical assessment from their physician. In fact, seldom will a veteran discuss the current level of his or her disability with a private physician before filing a claim for increased benefits. It is also true that the average veteran will not determine exactly what he or she must medically prove before filing a claim for increased benefits.

There is a way to improve the odds that the VA will approve your claim when filing a claim for increased benefits. First, you must know the exact rating code your disability is classified under. To do find this, you need to obtain a complete copy of your claim file. Law entitles you to complete set of the files the VA has on you. Once you have a copy of your claims file, find the *very last rating decision*. From this document, determine the four digit rating code assigned to your disability.

The last step in the process is to compose a statement on VA Form 21-4138 stating your intent to file a claim for increased benefits. Again, the statement should be short and to the point, covering the technical requirements of your claim. I would suggest something along these lines:

> Please accept this statement as a request for increased benefits for my service-connected lower back injury rated under rating code 5295. My orthopedic physician, Dr. Robert Young, after reviewing VA standards for a lumbosacral strain, finds that my condition is best rated under "severe at 40%." His letter of April 1, 1997, details his medical findings. Also enclosed is a sworn statement from my wife of 20 years whose lay observations report the difficulty I have in dealing with everyday tasks because of pain and loss of motion.

REOPENED CLAIM

A claim can be reopened after it has been adjudicated and previously denied. A claimant may reopen a claim either if he or she initially failed to appeal a VA decision within a year following the denial notice or (2) if his or her appeal was not granted. A claim may be reopened only on the grounds of new and material evidence or by claiming the VA committed a clear and unmistakable error. It is incredibly difficult to reverse the original decision of denial. To understand the mechanics and legal aspects of reopening claims, I suggest you obtain a copy of my book *Veterans Survival Guide: How to File and Collect on VA Claims*.

Rules that shape a winning claim action are briefly discussed as follows. A successful claimant must have a basic understanding of what is involved in the development of a claim. Nearly all the topics discussed below are examined in detail in later chapters.

A Documented Claim Is a Must

The VA will dismiss any claim action it perceives as not well documented. You have the duty to submit evidence sufficient to justify a belief by a fair and impartial individual that the claim is plausible or capable of substantiation. This means that you cannot just go into the VA with a claim application stating: "I have PTSD caused by what I experienced in Iraq." Simply claiming your medical condition is the result of an active service in Iraq will not qualify you as being disabled by PTSD. You must back it up with evidence.

As previously stated in chapter 4, there are three conditions that must be met. If your records support that you engaged in combat with the enemy, the first condition has been met.

Until you have met this first requirement, the law does not require the VA to assist you in developing your claim. To this end, you must know how to prove your claim. Failure to do so will result in a denial of your claim. If you stick it out, you'll be in for a three- to five-year battle establishing only one issue—that your claim was well grounded. Assuming you are successful in eventually proving your claim was well grounded, the VA will then go back to square one and look at your alleged injury based on all available evidence and decide if service connection is warranted. Should your claim be denied or underrated, you will have no other choice but to start the appeal process all over again, which means another three to five year wait. As you can see, a final decision on a hastily filed claim action could take a decade. The question you must ask yourself is, "Will I be alive when the claim runs its course?" Do it right the first time. Make certain your claim is well grounded and that there is evidence to support your contention that you were indeed injured or sickened while in the service.

No Record Equals No Claim

If you do not have copies of your active duty outpatient or inpatient medical records, you must obtain these. Outpatient medical records and military hospital records are maintained separately at the National Personnel Records Center in St. Louis, MO. Outpatient records are kept with your administrative and personnel records and inpatient records are stored in the hospital records section. When requesting a search for hospital records, you'll be asked to provide your full name, military serial number, the military unit your were assigned to at the time of hospitalization, the name and location of the hospital, the dates you were hospitalized, and the reason for the hospitalization.

Under the 1996 Memorandum of Understanding between the Department of Defense and the Department of Veterans Affairs, medical records of all military members retiring or separating after May 1, 1994, are transferred directly to the VA rather than to the National Personnel Records Center. The agreement calls for the military branch to forward medical records to the Department of Veterans Affairs Records Management Center, St. Louis, MO, for those members not initiating a claim. If the member initiates a claim during out-processing, his or her medical records will be transferred directly to the VA Regional Office closest to the veteran's future address.

How the VA Rates an Injury or Disease

When all the medical facts evidencing your claim have been gathered, the evidence is cross-referenced against *38 Code of Federal Regulations*, part 4, Schedule for Rating Disabilities. This section of the *CFR* lists the medical problems that VA rates as service connected.

Because this section of the 38 *CFR* has not been updated since 1945, there are no rating descriptions for many new disabling conditions. The rating board member makes an "analogous rating," which simply means he or she finds an injury or disease that is closely related. This decision-making process by a rating board member is highly subjective. A rating given under this procedure should be carefully scrutinized. You can recognize a rating for a disability that has not diagnostic code assigned to it by the last two numbers in a four digit rating code: 99.

Before you submit a claim for a particular medical problem, obtain a copy of 38 *CFR* part 4 and compare your medical condition to the rating schedule for that condition. The schedule will tell you what medical facts must be shown before the VA will grant service connection.

Testimonial Evidence Is a Must

To make sure you have probative evidence of an injury or disease, you must know how to prepare a sworn written statement to support your claim. The VA is quick to disregard "buddy letters" as evidence. However, a properly executed deposition giving a detailed explanation of pertinent facts from you, members of your family, fellow employees, employer, or former military comrades is vital, *relevant* evidence. Although they may not want to, the VA must give this type of evidence considerable weight. The VA can disregard your sworn statements only if they have hard, factual evidence to the contrary. You must learn how to construct these statements so they relate facts, not opinions or conjecture (see Donna Raz's statement in chapter 3 for a good example). The deposition must demonstrate how your medical condition affects your daily routine in the work place.

The First Weak Link: Adjudication

The working rules are translated from laws passed by Congress—they are not arbitrary rules that claims examiners and rating board members can create, ignore, or change at will. However, VA ROs, contrary to former Secretary Jessie Brown's belief, violate the law frequently.

Very few veterans are aware that their claim file must be reviewed and made part of the examination by the doctor. It is the duty of the senior claims examiner requesting the examination to ensure that the hospital or clinic has the file prior to the examination.

To ensure a just and fair decision on your claim, you must understand what the law requires of those rating the claim. Unless you are knowledgeable about what takes place during this process, it's very likely that your claim will be denied or, if granted, the award may be considerably less than what your disability justifies.

Willful Misconduct: Benefits Denied

Determining whether your alcohol or drug abuse was the result of willful misconduct is one of the first items a rating specialist will consider if you are claiming that your substance abuse is secondary to PTSD. The exception occurs when the VA can prove the facts were patently inconsistent with the evidence and the laws administrated by the Department of Veterans Affairs.

If your claim is denied on the basis of willful misconduct, the VA claims examiners must give you a detailed account of how they arrived at this conclusion. If their explanation does not discuss the evidence used and how they arrived at their decision, they are in violation of their own regulations. At this point, you should appeal the denial of benefits.

Presumption of Soundness: A Key Issue

The governing regulations pertaining to "presumption of soundness" are 38 *CFR* §3.304(b) and 38 *CFR* §3.305(b). Both regulations state that a veteran will be considered to have been in sound condition when examined, accepted, and enrolled for service, with exception made for the defects, infirmities, and disorders noted on the entrance examination. *When* the claimant entered the service is the difference between the two regulations. Regulation 38 *CFR* §3.304 (b) addresses those claims for veterans who served after January 1, 1947, whereas 38 *CFR* §3.305(b) covers claims for those who served prior to January 1, 1947. There is one other important difference between the two regulations. Individuals serving on active duty prior to January 1, 1947, have to have served on active duty six or more months before the presumption of soundness policy applies to their claim.

The law provides that any defects, infirmities, or disorders noted during the entry examination will not be considered service-related conditions unless they are aggravated by service. Both regulations stipulate that there must be clear and unmistakable evidence that demonstrates the injury or disease existed before entry into the service. A key point to remember is that only those medical conditions recorded on the entrance examination can be considered preexisting. An isolated reference in the medical file alleging a condition existed prior to service cannot be the sole bases for denial of benefits.

On several occasions the Court of Appeals for Veterans' Claims has addressed the issues of denial of benefits based on pre-existing medical conditions and pre-sumption of soundness. The case of *Parker v. Derwinski*[4] illustrates how the VA deviates from its own regulations in applying varying interpretations to the issue under consideration.

Mr. Parker sought to reopen his claim for disability benefits based on alleged vision deficiency caused by a hole in his left eye. The VA justified its denial of ser-vice connection because of the absence of any indication of trauma during active duty and an unsubstantiated statement by an army doctor referring to an alleged in-jury when Parker was nineteen years old. The VA concluded that this evidence was sufficient to rebut the presumption of soundness rule.

To prevail, the VA had to find that a preexisting injury or disease had been dem-onstrated by unmistakable evidence. The evidence did not support the VA position. They had two pieces of evidence: a statement from an army doctor alleging Mr. Parker injured his eye playing football at age nineteen and the fact that service medical records were silent as to an injury to the left eye. In its ruling, the court pointed out that the VA ignored Mr. Parker's sworn statement and the statements of several doctors in evi-dence. The court vacated the VA decision and remanded it back to the Regional Of-fice for readjudication.

This particular veteran's claim was handicapped by the fact that he waited ten years after leaving the service before filing his original claim for service connection. His initial claim was denied, and he filed no appeal. In 1987, after waiting another ten years, he tried to reopen his claim based on new and material evidence; this claim was promptly denied. Again, he did not appeal the denial. Each time he tried to reopen his claim, he included one new letter from a friend or doctor. In 1989, after receiving another denial to reopen his claim, he filed a timely appeal. It wasn't until 1991 that his appeal made its way to the Court of Appeals for Veterans Claims.

This case is an excellent example of how a claim can be dragged out for decades. When you file your claim, it's imperative that you *not* assume someone else (i.e., the VA) will gather the evidence to support your contentions. This is *your* job. If you do take the easy way out and only file an application with the hope the VA will gather the evidence, you will lose.

Chronic Diseases

In order to receive service-connection benefits, a chronic disease must manifest itself to a degree of 10% or more within one year of the date of separation from the service. However, there are several exceptions to this rule. If leprosy or tuberculosis develops at a 10% level of disability within three years, or multiple sclerosis within seven years, then service connection under this rule will be granted.[5]

The key word in this guideline is "manifest" and it is not synonymous with a diagnosis. If you can prove that during the year following separation the symptoms for the condition equate to a 10% rating, as stated in the Schedule for Rating Disabilities, then the disease will be considered a service-related medical problem. The forty-two diseases listed in 38 *CFR* §3.309(a) will be considered chronic under the presumptive rule:

- anemia, primary
- arteriosclerosis
- arthritis
- atrophy, progressive muscular
- brain hemorrhage
- brain thrombosis
- bronchiectasis
- calculi of the kidney, bladder, or gallbladder
- cardiovascular-renal disease including hypertension
- cirrhosis of liver
- coccidioidomycosis
- diabetes mellitus
- encephalitis lethargica residuals
- endocarditis (all forms of valvular heart disease)
- endocrinopathies
- epilepsies
- hansen's disease
- hodgkin's disease
- leukemia
- lupus erythematosus, systemic
- myasthenia gravis
- myelitis
- myocarditis
- nephritis
- other organic diseases of the nervous system
- osteitis deformans (Paget's disease)
- osteomalacia
- palsy, bulbar
- paralysis agitans
- psychoses
- purpura idiopathic, hemorrhagic

- raynaud's disease
- sarcoidosis
- scleroderma
- sclerosis, amyotrophic lateral
- sclerosis, multiple
- syringomyelia
- thromboangiitis obliterans (Buerger's disease)
- tuberculosis, active
- tumor malignant brain
- tumors, malignant, or of the brain or spinal cord or peripheral nerves
- ulcers, peptic (gastric or duodenal).

Tropical Diseases

Historically, the tropics have presented serious medical hazards for military members. Realizing this, Congress presumes service connection for sixteen diseases and resultant disorders. Also recognized is that treatment for many of these diseases could cause adjunct disabilities as a result of the therapy administered or as a preventive measure.

However, Congress also wrote into the law a rebuttal rule that the VA claims examiners must satisfy before presumptive service connection can be granted. The claim can be denied if the VA can show that the individual did not serve in a locality having a high incidence rate of the disease, or when the disease did not occur continuously in the local population. It can also be denied if the claimant separated from the service after the known incubation period for the tropical disease.

One of the sixteen diseases in this presumptive group is amebiasis, a disease that is generally characterized by dysentery with diarrhea, weakness, and prostration. The disease may be in remission for several years after exposure. When the patient does experiences the first symptom, it is often diagnosed as a stomach virus and treated accordingly.

When the patient doesn't respond to the standard treatment normally given for a stomach virus, the doctor usually orders a more serious study. At this point, the findings usually show the individual as being disabled by amoebas (microscopic parasites). The patient then learns from his doctor that his chronic condition is not found to be common where he lives, and he is also advised that the disease is not known to be a common health problem at his last duty station. He is told that it is common in the tropics—such as in Southeast Asia—and is acquired by ingesting food or drink containing encysted forms.

Then the patient recalls that just before his discharge, he was on temporary duty for one week in Saigon, South Vietnam. He and his friends made a tour of the local sights and ate and drank in local restaurants. A claim is filed and then is promptly denied by the VA on the basis of not being a well-grounded claim. The claimant's medical records do not establish treatment for the condition on active duty. His service records show he was never stationed in any tropical regions where the disease was prevalent. His records also establish he was discharged more than two years ago.

This is a winnable claim, but the claimant must properly develop it before filing a formal application. In this situation, file an informal claim to protect the date and serve notice to the VA that a service-connected disability claim will be forthcoming. (Detailed discussion related to various types of claim actions will be discussed in chapter 6.)

Three sections within 38 *CFR* part 3 govern the awarding of service connection for one of the sixteen tropical diseases presumed to be service connected if they manifest to a degree of 10% within a year of separating from the service. The sixteen diseases are identified in 38 *CFR* §3.309(b). Next, 38 *CFR* §3.307(a)(1)(4) requires a veteran to have served at least ninety days after December 31, 1946, and that the disease manifest to a degree of 10% or more within one year from the date of separation. The third condition outlined in 38 *CFR* §3.308(b) requires that a veteran who separated before January 1, 1947, serve at least six months on active duty before becoming eligible for presumptive service connection.

Combat-Related Injuries and Diseases

Official records or documents are not required to support your claim if you are a combat veteran and you file a claim for injuries or diseases that were incurred or aggravated *while* engaged in wartime operations against hostile forces. The VA is required to accept satisfactory lay or other evidence as the basis for the claim as long as the evidence is consistent with the circumstances, conditions, or hardships of such service.

This rule refers to combat with the enemy. Being assigned to a combat unit conducting tactical operations during a declared wartime, or during undeclared wartime engagements such as campaigns or expeditions supporting the United States or the United Nations for diplomatic purposes may not qualify for direct service connection. But the real problem is establishing direct service connection is when the disability is PTSD. An example of a situation where direct service connection does not apply would be if a vehicle mechanic were assigned to a forward area base and, while on guard duty, he and his friend are ambushed. His friend dies right next to him. The psychological trauma of witnessing a death under these circumstances would not qualify him for direct service connection. This veteran would have to prove he witnessed this death *and* he was on guard duty when the incident occurred.

Your sworn statement of the events surrounding the injury or illness is not sufficient as evidence of combat-related injuries. However, sworn statements from members of your unit are acceptable evidence in establishing the basis of a well-grounded claim when there are no medical records to support your claim. This is an extremely important rule for veterans who served in a combat zone. Proof of receiving the Purple Heart or Combat Infantry Badge can establish your presence in a combat zone. Obtaining a copy of the official unit history during the period when you were wounded or when you became ill is considered proof your claim is combat related.

In one special case, *Collette v. Brown,* the U.S. Court of Appeals for the Federal Circuit reversed the Court of Appeals for Veterans Claims on the issue of what a veteran must prove if he or she alleges combat injuries are the basis of a claim.[6] The Appeal Court held that the VA must accept the veteran's lay evidence (a statement that the injury or disease occurred in combat), unless proof shows the contrary. The only element the veteran has to show is that he or she engaged in combat with the enemy. This decision is absolutely binding on all VA Regional Offices.

Chapter 5: What Have We Learned?

1. Sworn statements are evidence.
2. Anything that happens to you on active duty is service related unless there is a wanton disregard for safety or you are involved in a felonious criminal act.
3. If your entrance physical examination is silent as to a medical condition existing prior to joining the service, then it is presumed that you were in perfect health when sworn in.
4. Make certain that when you are examined for compensation benefits the VA doctor has your claim folder and has reviewed it prior to the exam.
5. The VA must accept a combat veteran's explanation of the circumstances of his or her injury or disease unless solid evidence exists that rebuts the veteran's account of the facts.

Notes

1. White House press release.
2. VA Fact Sheet, 2002.
3. "Judge Chastises Regional Offices," American Legion Magazine, January–February 1995.
4. *Parker v. Derwinski*, 1 F. 522 (Vet. App. 1992).
5. 38 CFR, Part 4, Section 4.96.
6. *Collette v. Brown*, 82 F.3d 389 (Fed. Cir. 1996).

R ating a claim for PTSD benefits is governed by the instructions and policy found in these regulations, manuals, case law, general counsel opinions, and medical manuals:

- 38 *CFR* §3.304, §3.326, §3.327, and §3.340;
- 38 *CFR* §4.2, §4.7, §4.18, §4.16 §4.125, §4.126, and §4.129;
- "Adjudication Procedures," M21-1, part III, chapter 5, paragraph 5.14; and M21-1, part VI, chapter 11, paragraph 11.37;
- M21-1, part VI, paragraph 1.02 and 1.09, change 116, July 16, 2004;
- "Adjudication Procedures," M 21-1, chapter 1, "Physical Examinations, Social Surveys, and Field Examinations";
- *Diagnostic and Statistical Manual of Mental Disorders,* 4th edition, revised (DSM-IV-R).

It is important to read these references before you file a claim for PTSD. The information provided can help ensure your claim is well-developed and that the VA cannot be rebut the evidence. Protect yourself by making certain the claim is fully developed before submitting it. You do not want to get caught in the time warp known as the "Appeal Process."

VA manual M21-1, part VI, chapter 7, §7.46 opens with the following statement, "The issue of service connection for PTSD is the sole responsibility of the rating board at the local level." Now, because so many ratings are being decided by single member boards, under no circumstances can you afford to submit a claim for PTSD or, for that matter, any other claim that is not well supported by irrefutable evidence.

As previously stated, the VA has downgraded the job skill level for rating board members and further complicated the matter by placing people in these positions that have no formal training in medicine or law. The bottom line is: *if they don't understand it, they will deny the claim.*

If you read the decisions published on the Internet by the Board of Veterans' Appeals, you will immediately realize local ROs are not doing their job when it comes to developing and deciding issues using their regulations and manuals.[1] This is why it is essential that you understand what a senior claims examiner must do when the claim is being decided. If you do everything right, you will know where to address your disagreement if the claim is denied.

Components of Your PTSD Claim

FIRST ELEMENT: EVIDENCE OF A STRESSOR

How you organize your claim for PTSD depends on the facts and circumstances surrounding the traumatic event that caused the disorder. The evidence supporting the claim will require corroborating proof your diagnosis with PTSD is current at the time of application. The medical evidence must also show that these symptoms and treatment have been continuous for at least one month. The next question to be answered is was the stressor a combat event or was a noncombat-related psychological trauma the root cause of the disorder. The last major question your claim must answer is whether the onset of PTSD was immediate or a delayed reaction to the stressor. The basis of a delayed trauma must be fully explained by the examining physician.

The VA will deny your claim speedily if it is not supported by a clear-cut medical diagnosis of an active PTSD condition. Without a clear diagnosis that makes the connection between your military experiences and the current disorder, you will not have the basis for a well-grounded claim. There is an exception to this rule in that if you have been awarded one of the medals or awards refer to in VA manual M21-1, chapter 5, paragraph 5.14(b)(1) then the VA must accept your word that the PTSD event was the result of engaging in combat against the enemy (see chapter 4 for the full text of this section).

Linking the in-service incident to your current diagnosed condition has to be substantiated. The VA will not to accept a diagnosis of PTSD if the basis of the diagnosis by a mental health specialist was the veteran's uncorroborated account of the event. By producing corroborating evidence, such as sworn "buddy statements" or copies of military records, the examiner can state that, based on the records he reviewed, it is more likely than not that the in-service stressor occurred as you have related.

The U.S. Army Joint Services Environmental Support Group and the Commandant of the Marine Corps have archives that may provide proof of a stressor, which may in turn help a veteran's claim.[2] When soliciting information from these agencies, make certain to provide the following information:

+ full name;
+ VA claim number, if you have one;
+ social security number;
+ military service number;

- unit of assignment and its location at the time of the stressor incident (give complete military address);
- type, place, and date of the specific stressor incident claimed;
- the names of other individuals involved or aware of the incident;
- a detailed statement of the events that took place (as best as you can remember).

I would also suggest that you send your request for this information through your senator or congressional representative since government function must give legislative inquiries a priority response. Information from any federal agency is available to you under the provisions of the Freedom of Information Act.

SECOND ELEMENT: TYPES OF STRESSORS
Combat-Related Stress

If you claim your PTSD is based on actual combat with the enemy, the VA must accept your account of what happened as true. When the U.S. Court of Appeals for Veterans Claims decided *Zarycki v. Brown* and *West v. Brown*,[3] these cases made it clear when the claimant engaged in combat with the enemy and the alleged stressors are related to such combat, no further evidentiary development will be required by the VA. Your lay testimony will be satisfactory, so long as it is consistent with the conditions of combat service or hardships of such service.

First, let's assume your mental health specialist determined you have been suffering from PTSD for the past month. The next step is to determine if the stressors were related to combat. This can be established from service department records and sworn lay statements.[4] The records will confirm when you arrived and departed the combat zone, the military organization to which you were assigned, your combat military occupational specialty code (MOS), and combat medals and decorations awarded. Most importantly, the VA accepts the Purple Heart, combat action ribbons, or the Combat Infantry Badge as proof of engagement with the enemy.

Although the VA is required to accept a sworn credible statement from a combatant, some corroboration is still required in addition to the veteran's word. Part 38 of *CFR* §3.304(f) states in part, "If the claimed stressor is related to combat, service department evidence that the veteran engaged in combat or that the veteran was awarded the Purple Heart, Combat Infantryman Badge, or similar combat citations will be accepted, in the absence of evidence to the contrary, as conclusive evidence of the claimed in-service stressor."

When the claim is submitted, the evidence package attached to support your entitlement should include copies of orders and award letters, a certified copy of your DD-214, and copies of pertinent medical records and assessments that link your combat experiences to the current PTSD condition. Make the effort to get this information so you do not have to rely on the VA to try and develop corroboration that you were, in fact, in combat and that you are suffering from PTSD. There are several important reasons for taking this proactive step. First, it will shave months off the processing time required to decide your claim. Second, you will be in control, because you proved entitlement upon application. If the VA is going to deny the claim, claims examiners must prove (with hard evidence) your evidence is insufficient to grant benefits.

Noncombat-Related Stressors

The basic requirements in establishing a claim for PTSD benefits as a noncombatant are similar to those required for a combat-related diagnosis of PTSD. First, you must medically establish that you have been currently suffering from PTSD for at least one month. The primary difference between a claim based on a combat-induced stressor and that of a noncombat stressor is that in the latter, your sworn statement alone is not sufficient to establish the basis for a claim. Your statement regarding the cause of your PTSD must be supported by credible and corroborated evidence.

This does not mean that corroboration can only come from your service records. A sworn statement from individuals knowledgeable of the events that caused your stressor is acceptable evidence. A medical assessment from a mental health specialist is another example of corroborative evidence where the causes and effects of your in-service stressor are discussed in detail. Make certain the medical assessment by your doctor clearly states the root of your problem was traced back to a stressor that occurred in the service. As long as your service records do not contradict this type of evidence, the VA cannot deny your claim on the grounds that there was no proof in your service records to support the claim.[5]

One other important distinction made when the court ruled in *Doran V. Brown* was that a qualifying stressor must be based on an event. Mere service in a combat zone does not qualify as a stressor for PTSD. The court held, "It is the distressing event rather than the mere presence in a 'combat zone,' which may constitute a valid stressor for purposes of supporting a diagnosis of PTSD."

The Case of Robert E. Doran

The Court of Appeals for Veterans Claims gave veterans claiming PTSD based on noncombat-related stressors a leg up when it decided Robert Doran's case, *Doran v. Brown*. The court closed the door on one of the VA's most frequently used reasons for denying claims: "the absence of support in service records."[6]

Mr. Doran reopened his claim for psychoneurosis to include post-traumatic stress disorder in 1976, based on new and material evidence. However, it wasn't until August 1992 that his case made its way through the system to the court for the first time. He submitted medical evidence from the doctor who treated him for his neurosis and PTSD. He was also able to obtain lay statement from individuals who were knowledgeable of the circumstances of his stressors.

Mr. Doran claimed that during his active service (1950–1952), he was struck by lightning, which caused him to become unconsciousness and require resuscitation. The second stressor Mr. Doran cited was an encounter with a snake on an infiltration course. From the records available to the court, the evidence submitted in support of his claim was considered noncumulative, relevant to, and probative to the issue at hand. In other words, the evidence that Mr. Doran submitted was new, clarified the argument under appeal, and proved his claim. On August 7, 1992, the court issued a single-judge memorandum decision vacating the Board of Veterans' Appeals' November 28, 1990, denial of service connection and remanded it back to the VA for readjudication.

The court held that the "board focused only on evidence that tended to support the denial of service connection, ignored evidence in favor of the appellant's claim, and failed to provide reasons or basis for its findings and conclusions."[7] The order further stipulated that on remand, the board would adjudicate Mr. Doran's claim for service connection for PTSD, which was raised but never addressed.

On March 5, 1993, the Board of Veterans' Appeals (BVA) issued a decision in which it determined (1) the evidence received by the VA since the BVA denied entitlement for service connection for a psychoneurosis in September 1976 was both new and material and the claim for psychoneurosis to include PTSD would be reopened, (2) Mr. Doran's psychoneurosis preexisted active service and the sound condition at enlistment had been rebutted, (3) the psychoneurosis was not aggravated during service, and (4) service connection for PTSD was not warranted. Mr. Doran filed a timely appeal to the court.

One year later, on March 8, 1994, a three-judge panel heard Mr. Doran's appeal to the court. That portion of the court's discussion and decision concerning the aggravation of a preexisting psychoneurotic condition will not be addressed here as it is not pertinent to establishing service connection for PTSD.

The court found that the BVA's treatment of Mr. Doran's claim for PTSD highlighted the inconsistencies among the statute, the regulations, and the specific provisions of VA Adjudication Manual M21-1. The court gave a new definition to that section of the manual that required "service records must support the assertion that the veteran was subjected to a stressor of sufficient gravity to evoke symptoms (PTSD) in almost anyone."[8]

The court held that under the governing statutory and regulatory provisions regarding claims for service connection for PTSD, "if the claimed stressor is not combat-related, appellant's lay testimony regarding in service stressors is insufficient to establish the occurrence of the stressor and must be corroborated by credible supporting evidence." "*There is nothing in the stature or the regulations which provides that corroboration must and can only be found in service records.*"[9] Those service records that are available must not contradict the appellant's lay testimony concerning his noncombat stressor. *VA manuals cannot give out instructions that are contrary to the statute.*

For the second time the court vacated the VA decision to deny benefits. Mr. Doran's case was remanded with instruction to readjudicate his claim for PTSD and make certain a critical examination of all the evidence was conducted when justifying the decision. It is not known if the VA has readjudicated his claim for PTSD and granted the benefits, or whether the local rating board has continued to deny his claim, thus forcing him to continue with the appeal process.

THIRD ELEMENT: MEDICAL EVIDENCE

The third element of your PTSD claim is actually divided into two very distinct sub-elements. It is crucial that you become knowledgeable of the requirements set forth in the regulations and manuals for how these instructions must be implemented by senior claims examiners.

The first sub-element considered by rating board members is whether the medical evidence is in compliance with VA "Adjudication Procedures" M21-1, part VI, §7.46(b) which provides the minimum medical prerequisites to be rated as suffering from PTSD.

The second sub-element is those instructions detailed in VA medical manual IB11-56, "Physician's Guide for Disability Evaluations Examinations." Compensation and Pensions examiners are required to follow the procedures outlined in this manual to ensure the claimant's disability is properly evaluated. The results of the examination are used to determine if benefits will be awarded, and, if so, how much will be granted. How well the C&P physician does his or her job in evaluating the claimant's disabilities will make or break a veteran's claim.

Establishing Minimum Medical Standards

The adjudication manual M21-1, part VI, §7.46(b) mandates the information a VA psychiatric medical examination must provide before a rating decision can be rendered. The preface to §7.46 states, in part, "[I]n order for the rating board to make that decision, the *examining psychiatrist* must present a clear diagnosis showing a detailed history of the stressful events which are thought to have caused the condition and a full description of past and present symptoms."[10] (Italics added.) The psychiatrist's report must show that the claimant's experience was an event that is outside the range of usual human experience and would be markedly distressing to almost anyone. Examples would include a serious threat to one's own life or physical well-being; a serious threat or harm to one's children, spouse, or family member; sudden destruction to one's own home or community; or witnessing another person being killed or severely maimed as a result of an accident or physical violence.[11]

Next, the psychiatrist's report must demonstrate how the claimant relives the traumatic event in *one* of the four following ways:

- recurrent and intrusive distressing recollections of the event;
- recurrent distressing dreams of the event;
- sudden acting or feeling as if the traumatic event were recurring (including a sense of reliving the experience, illusions, hallucinations, and dissociate flashback episodes, even those that occur upon awakening or when intoxicated);
- intense psychological distress at exposure to events or occasions that symbolize or resemble an aspect of the traumatic event, including anniversaries of the trauma.

The examination must also address what the patient will do to avoid persistent stimuli associated with the trauma or note the presence of numbing of general responsiveness (not present before trauma), as indicated by at least *three* of the seven following conditions:

- efforts to avoid thoughts or feelings associated with the trauma;
- efforts to avoid activities or situations that cause recollections of the trauma;
- inability to recall an important aspect of the trauma (psychogenic amnesia);
- markedly diminished interest in significant activities;
- feeling of detachment or estrangement from others;
- restricted range of affect, for example, unable to have loving feelings;
- sense of foreshortened future, for example, does not expect to have a career, marriage, or children or a long life.

The evaluation must record at least *two* of the six persistent symptoms of increased arousal (not present before the trauma), from the following group of symptoms:

- difficulty falling or staying asleep;
- irritability or outbursts of anger;
- difficulty concentrating;
- hypervigilance;
- exaggerated startled response;
- physiologic reactivity upon exposure to events that symbolized or resemble an aspect of the traumatic event (e.g., a woman who was raped in an elevator breaks out in a sweat when entering any elevator).

The claimant must exhibit the symptoms of the disturbance (as described in the sub-paragraphs) for at least one month. If the onset of symptoms was at least six months after the trauma, the physician must specify the reason for the delayed trauma reaction. It's important to note at this time that the VA acknowledges that it might be years after the traumatic event before the disorder surfaces. However, the examining psychiatrist should comment on the present or absence of traumatic events and their relevance to the current symptoms. The veteran must provide to the examiner relevant, specific information concerning what happened, with as much detailed information as possible. Information about the event to provide includes the time (year, month, day), geographical location (corps, province, town, or other landmark feature such as a river or mountain), and names of others who may have been involved in the incident.

In the event the claim for PTSD is based on stressors such as rape, sexual assault, or sexual harassment, the rating board expects the C&P examiner to give the claimant an extensive psychiatric examination. The examining psychiatrist will elicit a detailed history of the stressful events that caused the condition and a full description of the past and present symptoms. VA adjudicators in general seem to not believe women who claim PTSD as a result of rape, sexual harassment, or sexual assault, unless there is a police report or hospital examination recording the event.

It is important to recognize that the statutes, regulations, and case law that govern the administrative conduct of the adjudication division have absolutely no control over the operation of the hospital and its duty toward patients or the examinee. The Veterans Benefits Administration has no legal authority to direct or dictate policy governing the activities of the hospital administration that conducts the C&P evaluations. A good analogy used to explain the relationship between these two organizations is to compare them to two Smith families, unrelated by blood, living on the same block. The Mr. Smith living at one end of the block cannot tell the Mr. Smith living at the other end of the block just how to cut his grass. If he tried, the second Mr. Smith would shoot back the "f word." Herein lies one of the major reasons why many veterans are so often denied benefits. The merit of the medical aspects of your claim is affected by the type of C&P examination you receive. This critical element is discussed in detail in chapter 7.

Developing a Winning Claim

The best way to maintain control throughout the entire claims process is to stay on the offensive. *Do not file* a claim until you know that the i's have been dotted and the t's have been crossed.

FIRST STEP
The first step in building a winning case is to file an informal claim. By doing so, the entitlement date is protected and you have up to one year to prepare your claim and

obtain all evidence necessary to prove entitlement. For our purposes, let's say that you sustained a traumatic war experience that has been diagnosed as post-traumatic stress disorder. The severity of the condition is characterized by your severe withdrawal from contact with other people, your inability to maintain steady employment, and thoughts of suicide, just to name some of the symptoms. Much of your physical ability is limited because of the PTSD.

SECOND STEP

Your next step is obtaining copies of all VA regulations, manuals, and pertinent case law that may relevant for your circumstances. Copies of VA regulations (38 *CFRs*) can be found in your local county law library or through the VA website. Copies of U.S. Court of Appeals for Veterans Claims decisions can also be found at a library (West's Veterans Appeals Reporter). The AMIE protocol can be found in chapter 7 and chapter 4 contains excerpts of many other regulations.

THIRD STEP

Third, arrange an appointment with your personal medical specialist and request an assessment of your condition. Make sure your doctor has a copy of 38 *CFR*, part IV regulation, "The AMIE Protocol Exam," copies of any service medical records, and a copy of any lay statements from people knowledgeable of the injury, disease, or condition. If others have treated you for these, obtain copies of these records.

If you do not have a specialist to work with, your local AMA chapter or hospital referral service will provide the names of doctors whose specialty covers your condition. To save yourself grief and unnecessary expenses, first determine if the doctor will give you a written assessment of the findings. If the doctor is not willing to put all findings in writing, tell him or her, "thank you, but without a written report, this evaluation would be totally useless for VA purposes."

FOURTH STEP

Your next step is to develop a lay statement to support the authenticity of your claim. Unless you file a claim within the first year following your separation, the VA has shown a history of denying benefits based solely on the fact that service medical records are silent as to your condition. All lay statements should be in the form of a sworn deposition so that these statements become evidence.

Remember, a statement from family or service friends will not be accepted as valid evidence if the statement is gives a medical opinion. A lay statement can give sworn testimony as to what was observed. It is important that the veteran give a sworn detailed statement as to what occurred, where he or was treated, and how often he or she was treated prior to filing the claim. Refer back to Sergeant Raz's sworn statement in chapter 3 to assist you in collecting your thoughts. If the injury occurred during combat with the enemy, then your statement alone is sufficient to establish service incurrence.

FIFTH STEP
The last step is to prepare all the supporting evidence to be appended to your claim. You are now ready to file your official claim and are prepared to take any scheduled C&P Exams within the next few months.

Chapter 6: What Have We Learned?

1. The VA must follow all its published rules. Failure to do so is an appealable action.
2. Each of the statutes, *CFRs*, and manuals are online by linking to the VA Home Page (www.va.gov) and search under Compensation and Pension Directives.
3. Your claim must have all three elements in order to qualify for service-connected PTSD.
4. The U.S. Army Joint Services Environmental Support Group or the Commandant of the Marine Corps are sources of obtaining records to substantiate your claim.
5. Always have your congressional representative or senator obtain these records on your behalf.
6. If at all possible, have a non-VA health provider evaluate your condition before filing a formal claim.
7. If you're claiming PTSD is caused by combat with the enemy, support it with a list of your medals and the corresponding citation that was given. Proving you were directly involved in combat will save you years of haggling with the VA.
8. PTSD-caused noncombat stressors is more difficult to pursue because you have the burden to prove the event did, in fact, occur and is responsible for your PTSD.
9. Reread the section "Establishing Minimum Medical Standards." You have to meet these standards in order move your claim along.
10. PTSD symptoms may first surface decades following the actual traumatic experience.
11. If service connection was denied and the claim met all the standards, *don't give up*. If Sgt. David Raz gave up, he wouldn't be rated 70% today. Go back and reread chapter 3, then appeal the denial of benefits.

Notes

1. The Board of Veterans Appeals' website allows you to search for decisions that may be favorable to your case: http://www.index.va.gov/search/va/index.jsp.
2. All service members (except marines) should write to: U.S. Army and Joint Services Environmental Support Group (ESG), Building 5089, Room 101, Stop #387, Fort Belvoir, VA, 22060. Inquires from marines should be addressed to Commandant, Headquarters U.S. Marines Corps, ATTN: MMRB-16, Quantico, VA, 22134-0001.
3. *Zarycki v. Brown*, 6 F. 91 (Vet. App. 1993); *West v. Brown*, 7 F. 70 (Vet. App. 1994).
4. Copies of the following documents can be obtained from the National Personnel Records Center (NPRC) by submitting form SF 180: orders assigning you to a combat unit (DD-214); copies of orders designating your MOS citations and orders awarding the Combat Infantry Badge; medals and awards reflecting hands-on combat duty.
5. See highlights of *Doran v. Brown*, 6 F.283 (Vet. App. 1994).
6. *Doran v. Brown*, 6 F. 283 (Vet. App. 1994).
7. Ibid.
8. Ibid.
9. Ibid.
10. Action Alert! If you were denied service connection for PTSD for any one or all of the items discussed in this portion of the chapter, it will pay to reopen your claim based on a clear and unmistakable error, provided you have not previously appealed the decision. VA Manual M21-1 §7.46 states the examination will be conducted by a psychiatrist. Case law requires that no examination should take place unless the examining physician has reviewed your complete case file at the time of the examination. The C&P evaluation report must conform to §7.46(b) regarding the information required by this paragraph. If the rating board did not comply with §7.46(d), return the examination as incomplete to the C&P examiner when the report failed to comply with §7.46(b).
11. APA, DSM-IV-R.

The Department of Veterans Affairs Health Administration has four primary functions: first, mandatory in-patient and out-patient treatment for service-related disabilities; second, treatment of non-service-related injuries and diseases based on the availability of medical services and patients' financial resources; third, conduct Compensation and Pension (C&P) examinations; and fourth, medical research.

The purpose of this chapter is to explain what the VA must do when they conduct a C&P examination for PTSD. Most importantly, you'll learn what to do if you are not given a *thorough and contemporaneous medical examination*, a phrase used often by the U.S. Court of Appeals for Veterans in cases involving flawed C&P examinations. Millions of veterans are cheated out of lawful benefits because of flawed C&P examinations and the flawed interpretation of these examinations by senior claims examiners who have neither medical nor legal training nor experience.

VA Health Administration

Before focusing on the VA's responsibility to administer C&P examinations, a general discussion of the overall operation of the VA Heath Administration is in order. During the latter part of 1997, VA medical service came under the scrutiny of both Congress and the public because of abusive management styles, condoning sexual harassment of patients and employees, many unnecessary deaths of veterans in VA medical facilities, and congressional pressure to cut operating costs and reduce services. During a nineteen-month period (mid-1997 to late 1998) more than three thousand medical mistakes were documented that resulted in more than seven hundred deaths.[1]

Here are some of the newspaper headlines that captured the public's attention during 1997 and weakened the trust and confidence in VA medical care:

- Deaths, Federal Probe Surface at VA Centers
- Disabled VA Doctor's Assignment Criticized, Managed Care?
- VA Hospital Leads Nation in Settlements
- VA Managers Grilled on Patient Deaths
- Families Ask VA: Did You Treat Our Loved Ones Properly?

- VA Focus on Fatal Errors
- House to Review Harassment at VA
- Under Fire, VA Administrator Leaves
- Deaths Haunt Miami VA Hospital
- Troubles at Small VA Hospital Mirror Agency Overall
- Lawsuit Sparks New Investigation of VA Doctor[2]

Contradicting VA Hoopla

To create a medical environment where the quality of care is influenced primarily by budget considerations is a wanton disregard of the intent of the laws authorizing medical care of veterans. Every effort of VA healthcare management strives to cut operational costs without any concern for the end effect on patients. Employing physicians who must only meet minimum standards to practice medicine has generated great savings. In the private sector, if a doctor moves from New York to Florida, he or she must be relicensed in Florida in order to practice medicine. However, not so with the VA: *U.S. Code Title 38* requires only that a doctor graduate from a medical school approved by the Secretary (which could be anywhere in the world); complete an internship satisfactory to the Secretary (no standards prescribed in the law); and obtain a one-time license to practice medicine, surgery, or osteopathy *in any state and in any field*, without board certification and postgraduate training in his or her field to qualify for VA employment.[3] Over the years the press has reported cases where a state's medical board revokes a doctor's license and the doctor now practices medicine for the VA in another state without having to be relicensed.

Beyond the requirements listed above, there are no other professional standards demanded of VA doctors. The plus side of requiring only minimum professional experience is the VA can pay them less than physicians who are diplomats of their medical specialty. The law also allows VA hospitals to hire doctors under fee or part-time arrangements. They are also allowed to hire interns, doctors in residency, and physician's assistants.

Using Part-time and Fee-Based Physicians

Many VA hospitals hire retired doctors with only a general medical background to conduct C&P examinations and to perform other medical services that would normally require the skills of a specialist. The VAMC Bay Pines, Florida, use fee-based doctors along with physician's assistants to conduct C&P exams.

The danger in using fee-basis or part-time, nonspecialist physicians for a veteran's C&P examination is best demonstrated by a case I worked on. An eighty-year-old, retired physician conducted C&P and psychiatric examinations under a fee-based arrangement with the VA. The VA profited by this situation because many veterans with psychiatric disorders were not properly evaluated and thus were denied benefits or given benefits at a rate less than entitled. This doctor's fees were inexpensive when compared to full-time, board-certified psychiatrists whose fees are earned based on education and experience. Because of the flawed examination administered by this doctor, I spent years appealing before I recaptured my client's 100% total disability rating. This long delay was also caused by the stubbornness of the local rating boards in acknowledging that the veteran's initial psychiatric examination had been flawed.

The Fee Based Program functions very much like piecework jobs. VA doctors are paid for a set number of examinations and receive a flat-rate fee as compensation. This program is, without a doubt, one of the greatest disservices burdening veterans in their quest for legitimate claims resolution.

Veterans Healthcare Reform Act of 1996

In September 1996, the VA Health Administration announced another new healthcare strategy that discreetly further distanced itself from promises made for medical care to veterans who served their country. Veterans seeking medical care after October 1998 must apply annually for enrollment in the VA healthcare program at which time they will be assigned to one of eight priority groups. Failure to apply will make the veteran ineligible to receive medical treatment. The only exceptions to this policy are for veterans rated by the VA as having a service-connected disability of 50% or more, veterans discharged or separated from the service less than one year ago with a compensable disability, or veterans seeking care from the VA for only a service-connected disability. The group to which you are assigned will determine exactly what care you will receive; that is, veterans in one group receive the best care while veterans in another group receive no care. This categorization limits medical support to a very large, aging veteran population. Bureaucrats will never gain the kind of brownie points necessary to enjoy the rewards of a Republican politician unless they can cut the operating costs of the VA so the money can be spent on other important presidential initiatives.

Ironically, the House Committee on Veterans Affairs released a statement on September 30, 1996, to announce the new H.R. 3118—the Veterans' Health Care Eligibility Reform Act of 1996—a bill that specifically addresses the psychiatric needs of veterans. The press release says, in part:

> This veterans' health care bill would help streamline and strengthen the VA health care system by expanding, updating, and simplifying many outdated rules on eligibility for VA medical care. The bill would also substantially expand veterans' eligibility to receive treatment on an outpatient basis.

This reform would, for the first time, establish a "medical need" as the sole test for veterans who enroll for care with VA.

H.R. 3118 recognizes the important role of VA psychiatric care; more than 50 % of all eligible veterans who suffer from severe mental illness rely on VA for care. Among its provisions, the bill would authorize VA to establish for the first time, centers for excellence combining education, research, and clinical care of the severely mentally ill. (Italics added.)

You should be aware of another feature of this new healthcare program: the veteran's eligibility status will be evaluated annually by the primary care center to determine if he or she will remain in the current priority group, be assigned to a lower priority group, or be terminated from the program. For example, let's assume you are assigned to Priority Group 2 when first enrolled because you have a 30% service-connected disability. However, the VA rating board recently reduced your rating to 0% based on their interpretation of the results from a recent C&P examination. You are now transferred to Priority Group 6. This translates to continued priority care for your service-related condition. Any other medical problems will be treated at the lowest level of care offered.

Now that we have explored the structure of the VA and the relevant, governing legislation, it's time to consider the most important component in determining your eligibility for benefits: the Compensation and Pension Examination.

Compensation and Pension Examination

Almost all service-connected benefits extended to veterans rely on some degree of disability that was incurred in the service, aggravated in the service, or resulted from treatment in a VA facility by VA medical staff. The claim process for service connection requires the VA to obtain original service medical records, medical records from VA treatment centers (hospitals or clinics), copies of private physician's records, and hospital records before deciding the merits of the claim.

The *Code of Federal Regulations*, 38 §3.326(a) states that where a reasonable probability of a valid claim is indicated, a Department of Veterans Affairs examination will be authorized. However, the regulation also permits the rating board to decide the claim based on the findings of a private physician if the report meets certain standards. The specialist's report must include clinical manifestations and substantiation of diagnosis by findings of diagnostic techniques generally accepted by the medical authorities. Pathological studies, X-rays, and laboratory tests must be part of your specialist's assessment.

If the records are not sufficient to determine the current degree of disability or if the rating board elects not to accept your specialist's report for any reason, you will be scheduled for what is known as a C&P Examination. Herein lies a major unfairness to veterans.

The level of medical expertise of the examining physician is left to the discretion of the medical service being tasked. In my thirteen years working with veterans as an advocate, I don't recall a single case where a doctor board-certified for the condition being evaluated examined the veteran. All C&P examinations were administered by non–VA staff doctors who were recruited from the ranks of retired doctors. Almost all of the doctors I checked through the AMA Headquarters in Chicago were identified as family or general practitioners. A while back, using a veterans' bulletins board, I asked if it was a common practice throughout the United States for veterans to be examined by these fee-based general practitioners. The veterans' responses were not surprising: C&P examinations by nonspecialist doctors was a common practice of all VA Medical Centers.

The only time a general practitioner is not supposed to be used is when an appeal is remanded back with instructions that a board-certified specialist examine the claimant. VA manual M21-1[4] mandates this procedure be followed, yet the VA medical center will assign a variety of medical personnel; in many cases, the assignment goes to the same doctor who did the initial evaluation. I've yet to see a document in a claimant file noting the rating board returned the examination mandating the medical center assign a board-certified specialist.

This is why it's important for you to know the medical specialty of the physician who conducts your exam; it's the basis for an appeal if benefits are denied. The court has held many times that the VA has a duty to provide you with a thorough and contemporaneous examination. When you have a complex medical problem and a general practitioner examines you, a warning should sound for you.

Let me tell you of one incident to drive home the point. I was involved in a case where the veteran was completely disabled by Buerger's Disease. A part-time, general practitioner reported he did not agree with the findings of two well-known cardiologists, and the rating board denied the veteran's claim, agreeing therefore with the least capable physician. After six years and several trips to the BVA, the claim was granted. The veteran received a check for $88,000 in back benefits. The saddest part about the veteran's story is that he died within a year of being determined 100% disabled.

The Protocol for C&P Examinations

The process starts when a claim is filed for any benefit involving a disability or disease that was incurred in the service. Your claim and medical evidence is forwarded to the adjudication division where the medical evidence attached to your claim and service medical records are reviewed. By law, the rating board can rate your claim on this evidence alone if deemed adequate for rating purposes.

As discussed previously, the first hurdle that you must jump is the claim must be recognized as *well founded*. Assuming the claim meets this standard, the law mandates that the VA has a duty to assist the veteran from this point forward. If the rating board cannot make a rating based on the medical evidence submitted with the claim and the service medical records, the rater must request a C&P examination from a VA medical facility. The veteran should be scheduled for a C&P Exam by the medical facility closest to his or her home.

It is the rating board that tells the C&P Section medically what kind of examination to conduct. The exam request is then forwarded to the local VAMC electronically through the Automated Medical Information Exchange (AMIE). In most cases the rating board orders only a general evaluation with no specific requests for the veteran to see a specialist.

Even if the rating board requested a specialty examination, the hospital is not obligated to assign a specialist. Hospital personnel have complete freedom to assign whomever they choose. Through the years, I have seen them assign only fee-basis doctors or student residents from a local medical school to evaluate complex medical problems claimed by a veteran.

The *Code of Federal Regulations* 38 §4.2, "Interpretation of an Examination Report" requires the rating specialist to return the examination report when the diagnosis is not supported by the findings or if the examination report does not contain sufficient details. Rating boards seldom, if ever, return C&P examinations unless the veteran or the advocate has pointed out upon appeal that the examination was inadequate and thus flawed. Rating boards often deny benefits even when the exam protocol fails to follow the examining procedures outlined in the *C&P Service Clinician's Guide* (2002). I've never seen a rating board member study the results of a C&P Exam to ensure that the report submitted was in full compliance with the VA Manuals and Regulations. One reason for this is that the rating board members' shallow level of understanding of medicine is not sufficient for them to detect the flawed nature of the examination. If you looked at the remand and reversal rate of appeals reviewed by the Board of Veterans' Appeals (between 70% and 80% nationwide) you would see that rating boards are extremely deficient in the interpretation and application of the concepts related to law and medicine.

AMIE C&P Examination Program

The AMIE system is a multipurpose electronic system created to share administrative information between medical centers, outpatient clinics, and Regional Offices. The C&P Examination Program is a program within AMIE that allows ROs to electronically transmit examination requests to medical centers. After the medical center prints the requests and schedules specific examinations, standardized examination worksheets are printed. The printed request and worksheet now become the official record between the RO and medical center.

Obtaining copies of the records generated during the examination process is absolutely essential should you have to go head-to-head with the VA to dispute a decision. Following, briefly, are the steps of the program:

- The RO clerk electronically inputs the request for a C&P Exam to the VAMC.
- Upon receipt of the request, the medical center clerk schedules the exam.
- Worksheets are printed and the examination is scheduled.
- Using the printed worksheets, the examiner conducts the examination.
- The examiner dictates the report using the worksheet format.
- The transcriber enters the results into the system and routes a printed copy to the physician for review and signature.
- The examination report is electronically dispatched to the RO.
- The report is printed by the RO clerk and forwarded to the rating board for action.

A copy of the following records should be requested from the RO:

- the initial request for C&P examination transmitted to the medical facility;
- a copy of the doctor's report furnished to the RO; and
- a copy of any lab reports, X-rays, and special tests performed and sent to the RO.

From the VA medical facility performing the C&P examination, you'll need:

- a copy of the worksheet used by the examining physician;
- a copy of the dictated report of the examination;
- a copy of all tests results, radiological reports, and lab results; and
- a statement of the physician's qualifications.

AMIE's PTSD Protocol Examination

The eleven-page document shown in figure 7.1 is the actual worksheet used by C&P examiners when evaluating a veteran for PTSD. Study it! Know exactly what they should be exploring during the examination. Once the report is dictated and transmitted to the RO, immediately obtain a copy from the medical center. Compare the report to the protocol outlined to determine if every item was, in fact, covered. Look for any variation between your testimony and what was reported to the RO. Also keep track of how long the interview lasted. If the VA failed to do the job correctly, you have grounds for an appeal.

Fig. 7.1

Initial Evaluation for Post-Traumatic Stress Disorder (PTSD)

0910 Worksheet

Name: SSN:

Date of Exam: C-number:

Place of Exam:

The following health care providers can perform initial examinations for PTSD.
a board certified psychiatrist;
a licensed psychologist;
a psychiatry resident under close supervision of an attending psychiatrist or
psychologist; or
a psychology intern under close supervision of an attending psychiatrist or
psychologist.

A. Identifying Information

- age
- ethnic background
- era of military service
- reason for referral (original exam to establish PTSD diagnosis and related psychosocial impairment; reevaluation of status of existing service-connected PTSD condition)

B. Sources of Information

- records reviewed (C-file, DD-214, medical records, other documentation)
- review of social-industrial survey completed by social worker
- statements from collaterals
- administration of psychometric tests and questionnaires (identify here)

C. Review of Medical Records

1. Past Medical History:

   a. Previous hospitalizations and outpatient care.
   b. Complete medical history is required, including history since discharge from military service.
   c. Review of Claims Folder is required on initial exams to establish or rule out the diagnosis.

2. Present Medical History - over the past one year.

    a. Frequency, severity and duration of medical and psychiatric symptoms.
    b. Length of remissions, to include capacity for adjustment during periods of remissions.

D. Examination (Objective Findings)

Address each of the following and fully describe:

History (Subjective Complaints):
Comment on:

Pre-Military History (refer to social-industrial survey if completed)

- describe family structure and environment where raised (identify constellation of family members and quality of relationships)
- quality of peer relationships and social adjustment (e.g., activities, achievements, athletic and/or extracurricular involvement, sexual involvements, etc.)
- education obtained and performance in school
- employment
- legal infractions
- delinquency or behavior conduct disturbances
- substance use patterns
- significant medical problems and treatments obtained
- family psychiatric history
- exposure to traumatic stressors (see CAPS trauma assessment checklist)
- summary assessment of psychosocial adjustment and progression through developmental milestones (performance in employment or schooling, routine responsibilities of self-care, family role functioning, physical health, social/interpersonal relationships, recreation/leisure pursuits).

Military History

- branch of service (enlisted or drafted)
- dates of service
- dates and location of war zone duty and number of months stationed in war zone
- Military Occupational Specialty (describe nature and duration of job(s) in war zone

- highest rank obtained during service (rank at discharge if different)
- type of discharge from military
- describe routine combat stressors veterans was exposed to (refer to Combat Scale)
- combat wounds sustained (describe)
- clearly describe specific stressor event(s) veteran considered particularly traumatic. Clearly describe the stressor, particularly if the stressor is a type of personal assault, including sexual assault. Provide information, with examples, if possible.
- indicate overall level of traumatic stress exposure (high, moderate, low) based on frequency and severity of incident exposure (refer to trauma assessment scale scores described in Appendix B).
- citations or medals received
- disciplinary infractions or other adjustment problems during military service.

NOTE: Service connection for post-traumatic stress disorder (PTSD) requires medical evidence establishing a diagnosis of the condition that conforms to the diagnostic criteria of DSM-IV, credible supporting evidence that the claimed in-service stressor actually occurred, and a link, established by medical evidence, between current symptomatology and the claimed in-service stressor. It is the responsibility of the examiner to indicate the traumatic stressor leading to PTSD, if he or she makes the diagnosis of PTSD. *Crucial in this description are specific details of the stressor, with names, dates, and places linked to the stressor, so that the rating specialist can confirm that the cited stressor occurred during active duty.*

A diagnosis of PTSD cannot be adequately documented or ruled out without obtaining a detailed military history and reviewing the claims folder. This means that initial review of the folder prior to examination, the history and examination itself, and the dictation for an examination initially establishing PTSD will often require more time than for examinations of other disorders. Ninety minutes to two hours on an initial exam is normal.

Post-military Trauma History (refer to social-industrial survey if completed)

- describe post-military traumatic events (see CAPS trauma assessment checklist)

- describe psychosocial consequences of post-military trauma exposure(s) (treatment received, disruption to work, adverse health consequences)

  Post-military Psychosocial Adjustment (refer to social-industrial survey if completed), legal history (DWIs, arrests, time spent in jail)

- educational accomplishment
- employment history (describe periods of employment and reasons)
- marital and family relationships (including quality of relationships with children)
- degree and quality of social relationships
- activities and leisure pursuits
- problematic substance abuse (lifetime and current)
- significant medical disorders (resulting pain or disability; current medications)
- treatment history for significant medical conditions (including hospitalizations)
- history of inpatient and/or outpatient psychiatric care (dates and conditions treated)
- history of assaultiveness
- history of suicide attempts
- summary statement of current psychosocial functional status (performance in employment or schooling, routine responsibilities of self-care, family role functioning, physical health, social/interpersonal relationships, recreation/leisure pursuits)

E. Mental Status Examination

Conduct a brief mental status examination aimed at screening for DSM-IV mental disorders. Describe and fully explain the existence, frequency and extent of the following signs and symptoms, or any others present, and relate how they interfere with employment and social functioning:

- impairment of thought process or communication
- delusions, hallucinations and their persistence
- eye contact, interaction in session, and inappropriate behavior cited with examples
- suicidal or homicidal thoughts, ideations or plans or intent
- ability to maintain minimal personal hygiene and other basic activities of daily living

- orientation to person, place and time
- memory loss, or impairment (both short and long-term)
- obsessive or ritualistic behavior which interferes with routine activities and describe any found
- rate and flow of speech and note any irrelevant, illogical, or obscure speech patterns and whether constant or intermittent
- panic attacks noting the severity, duration, frequency and effect on independent functioning and whether clinically observed or good evidence of prior clinical or equivalent observation is shown
- depression, depressed mood or anxiety
- impaired impulse control and its effect on motivation or mood
- sleep impairment and describe extent it interferes with daytime activities

- other disorders or symptoms and the extent they interfere with activities, particularly:
  - mood disorders (especially major depression and dysthymia)
  - substance use disorders (especially alcohol use disorders)
  - anxiety disorders (especially panic disorder, obsessive-compulsive disorder, generalized anxiety disorder)
  - somatoform disorders
  - personality disorders (especially antisocial personality disorder and borderline personality disorder)

Specify onset and duration of symptoms as acute, chronic, or with delayed onset.

F. Assessment of PTSD

- State whether or not the veteran meets the DSM-IV stressor criterion.
- Identify behavioral, cognitive, social, affective, or somatic change veteran attributes to stress exposure.
- Describe specific PTSD symptoms present (symptoms of trauma re-experiencing, avoidance/numbing, heightened physiological arousal, and associated features [e.g., disillusionment and demoralization]).
- Specify onset, duration, typical frequency, and severity of symptoms.

G. Psychometric Testing Results

- Provide psychological testing if deemed necessary.
- Provide specific evaluation information required by the rating board or on a BVA Remand.
- Comment on validity of psychological test results.
- Provide scores for PTSD psychometric assessments administered.
- State whether PTSD psychometric measures are consistent or inconsistent with a diagnosis of PTSD, based on normative data and established "cutting scores" (cutting scores that are consistent with or supportive of a PTSD diagnosis are as follows: PCL $\geq$ 50; Mississippi Scale $\geq$ 107; MMPI PTSD subscale a score > 28; MMPI code type: 2-8 or 2-7-8).
- State degree of severity of PTSD symptoms based on psychometric data (mild, moderate, or severe).
- Describe findings from psychological tests measuring problems other than PTSD (MMPI, etc.).

H. Diagnosis

1. The Diagnosis must conform to DSM-IV and be supported by the findings on the examination report.
2. If there are multiple mental disorders, delineate to the extent possible the symptoms associated with each and a discussion of relationship.
3. Evaluation is based on the effects of the signs and symptoms on occupational and social functioning.

NOTE: VA is prohibited by statute, 38 U.S.C. 1110, from paying compensation for a disability that is a result of the veteran's own ALCOHOL OR DRUG ABUSE. However, when a veteran's alcohol or drug abuse disability is secondary to or is caused or aggravated by a primary service-connected disorder, the veteran may be entitled to compensation. See *Allen v. Principi*, 237 F.3d 1368, 1381 (Fed. Cir. 2001). Therefore, it is important to determine the relationship, if any, between a service-connected disorder and a disability resulting from the veteran's alcohol or drug abuse. Unless alcohol or drug abuse is secondary to or is caused or aggravated by another mental disorder, you should separate, to the extent possible, the effects of the alcohol or drug abuse from the effects of the other mental disorder(s). If it is not possible to separate the effects in such cases, please explain why.

I. Diagnostic Status

- Axis I disorders
- Axis II disorders
- Axis III disorders
- Axis IV (psychosocial and environmental problems)
- Axis V (GAF score - current)

J. Global Assessment of Functioning (GAF)

NOTE: The complete multi-axial format as specified by DSM-IV may be required by BVA Remand or specifically requested by the rating specialist. If so, include the GAF score and note whether it refers to current functioning. A BVA Remand may also request, in addition to an overall GAF score, that a separate GAF score be provided for each mental disorder present when there are multiple Axis I or Axis II diagnoses and not all are service-connected. If separate GAF scores can be given, an explanation and discussion of the rationale is needed. If it is not possible, an explanation as to why not is needed.

DSM-IV is only for application from 11/7/96 on. Therefore, when applicable, note whether the diagnosis of PTSD was supportable under DSM-III-R prior to that date. (Attach copies of relevant DSM-III-R sections.)

K. Capacity to Manage Financial Affairs

Mental competency, for VA benefits purposes, refers only to the ability of the veteran to manage VA benefit payments in his or her own best interest, and not to any other subject. Mental incompetency, for VA benefits purposes, means that the veteran, because of injury or disease, is not capable of managing benefit payments in his or her best interest. In order to assist raters in making a legal determination as to competency, please address the following:

What is the impact of injury or disease on the veteran's ability to manage his or her financial affairs, including consideration of such things as knowing the amount of his or her VA benefit payment, knowing the amounts and types of bills owed monthly, and handling the payment prudently? Does the veteran handle the money and pay the bills himself or herself?

Based on your examination, do you believe that the veteran is capable of managing his or her financial affairs? Please provide examples to support your conclusion.

If you believe a Social Work Service assessment is needed before you can give your opinion on the veteran's ability to manage his or her financial affairs, please explain why.

L. Other Opinion

Furnish any other specific opinion requested by the rating board or BVA remand (furnish the complete rationale and citation of medical texts or treatise supporting opinion, if medical literature review was undertaken). If the requested opinion is medically not ascertainable on exam or testing, please state why. If the requested opinion can not be expressed without resorting to speculation or making improbable assumptions, say so, and explain why. If the opinion asks " ... is it at least as likely as not ... ", fully explain the clinical findings and rationale for the opinion.

M. Integrated Summary and Conclusions

- Describe changes in psychosocial functional status and quality of life following trauma exposure (performance in employment or schooling, routine responsibilities of self-care, family role functioning, physical health, social/ interpersonal relationships, recreation/leisure pursuits).
- Describe linkage between PTSD symptoms and afore-mentioned changes in impairment in functional status and quality of life. Particularly in cases where a veteran is unemployed, specific details about the effects of PTSD and its symptoms on employment are especially important.
- If possible, describe extent to which disorders other than PTSD (e.g., substance use disorders) are independently responsible for impairment in psychosocial adjustment and quality of life. If this is not possible, explain why (e.g., substance use had onset after PTSD and clearly is a means of coping with PTSD symptoms).
- If possible, describe pre-trauma risk factors or characteristics than may have rendered the veteran vulnerable to develop-ing PTSD subsequent to trauma exposure.
- If possible, state prognosis for improvement of psychiatric condition and impairments in functional status.
- Comment on whether veteran is capable of managing his or her financial affairs.

Include your name; your credentials (i.e., a board certified psychiatrist, a licensed psychologist, a psychiatry resident or a psychology intern); and circumstances under which you performed the examination, if applicable (i.e., under the close supervision of an attending psychiatrist or psychologist); include name of supervising psychiatrist or psychologist.

Signature: Date:

Signature of Supervising psychiatrist or psychologist: Date:

Completeness of Reports

The examining physician is responsible for recording a complete and detailed report, including correct diagnosis analysis of the disabling condition and a description of the effects of the disability on the veteran's ordinary activity. The correct diagnosis is of great importance. The reports should include the clinical and laboratory findings as well as all other evidence that will substantiate the diagnosis and severity of the disability.

The recorded evidence of exact findings is just as important as the actual diagnosis itself in meeting the needs of a rating board member. Similarly, the findings and clinical evidence demonstrating the severity of the disability should be reported because in most claim actions for compensation benefits, the rating board member never sees the veteran. Clarity of description, legibility of notes, accuracy of dates, identification of normal ranges for tests reported and other details are crucial.

You should obtain a copy of the C&P examination and carefully review it to make certain the C&P examiner did, in fact, convey this detailed information in the report. If any information is missing, the rating board member is required under 38 *CFR* §4.2 to return the examination report as inadequate for evaluation purposes. However, I assure you, that rating board members do not routinely return C&P examination results unless the claimant states concern that benefits were denied because the report was inadequate.

Scope of the Examination

A request for a C&P examination from a rating board member will list all service connected disabilities, active, static, or alleged. It has been the practice of rating boards to ask only for a general medical examination instead of a specific examination directly related to the conditions being claimed. The manual states the "scope of the examination should be broad enough to cover all diseases, injuries and residuals, which are alleged by the veteran." But examinations should be made by a specialist; that is, when a patient has a heart condition, a cardiologist, not a nurse practitioner, should conduct the examination. In *Irby v. Brown*, the court held that the VA failed in its duty to assist by failing to order a thorough and contemporaneous psychiatric examination (specialty examination) and, as such, the report did not give a specific finding.[5]

The way the system works, if you have a serious back disorder with radiating pain, for example, a general practitioner will most likely evaluate you instead of an orthopedist or neurologist. Although this system is an economical way of containing the cost of care, you have the right to receive evaluations from specialists. Any lesser alternative is a breach of the doctrine decreed by this country to veterans who became disabled while serving the interest of the country.

If your claim was denied based on a C&P examination administered by a fee-based general practitioner, file a Notice of Disagreement (NOD), citing that the VA failed in its duty to assist by not providing a thorough and contemporaneous examination. In addition, you should cite either *Sklar v. Brown* or *Irby v. Brown,* whichever is most applicable.[6] Make certain that you state very clearly the reasons why the C&P examination was flawed and why either case law is applicable.

Severity of Disability

When reporting the findings of a C&P examination, the *Clinician's Guide* emphasizes that "the essential duty of the examining physician is to record a full, clear report of the medical and industrial history, the symptomatology and physical findings."[7] The purpose of the C&P report is to permit a rating board member to compare the medical findings reported by the examining physician with the disability percentage evaluations contained in the rating schedule.

For a client who intended to obtain a medical assessment from a private specialist of his choice, I always made a copy of the rating schedule for the private doctor. This provided the framework for the private specialist's report to be equated to the VA rating schedule. Thus, if the private examination report, supported by solid medical evidence, determined the veteran was 60% disabled and the VA rated the claim at 40% disabling based only on its own unsubstantiated conclusions, the veteran was on solid ground with a winnable appeal.

Review of the Claim Folder

The law requires that the veteran's claim file will be available to the C&P examiner and must be reviewed by the examiner prior to the examination. *This is one of the most important regulations that is violated and ignored by C&P physicians and rating board members alike.* The court and BVA have remanded case after case back to local ROs because they refuse to follow this policy, thus violating the veteran's right to a fair decision.

If the claim file is not present when you are examined, or if the examining physician has not read the file prior to the examination, grounds exist to appeal the denial of any benefit sought. If you do not see your claim file when being examined, ask the attending physician, "Do you have my claim file?" If you see the file, ask the doctor, "Have you read the claim file in its entirety?" If the answer is no to either question, the local RO should be advised immediately in writing that you did not receive a fair and contemporaneous examination because the examiner did not have your file present or was not aware of your case medical history. *Make a copy of your letter and send it by certified mail with a return receipt requested.*

Taking the Examination

Once you are scheduled for a C&P examination, you must comply with the order and report to the medical center or clinic or risk denial of benefits.[8] However, if the condition you are being evaluated for is cyclical—having inactive and active stages—and in remission at the time of your examination, you must contact the medical center and reschedule so that you can be evaluated and observed by a physician when the condition is active. Failure of the VA to evaluate your condition during an active stage is grounds for a reversal if the claim is denied.[9]

Medical examiners assigned to the C&P unit are notorious for sometimes spending only five to twenty minutes with a patient. There also exists the possibility, as previously discussed, that the evaluation will be flawed because the examination was all or in most part performed by someone other than the highest qualified doctor. The VA is notorious for substituting nurse practitioners or physician assistants to conduct C&P examinations. I speak from experience. I had an unqualified examiner whom the rating board really loved. During my C&P examination, she concluded that my heart conditions could not be considered service related because no professional medical studies had been published to substantiate my claim. She failed to read my file as she was supposed to. My file contained two board-certified cardiologists and one primary care physician statement concluding that my air force medical records did in fact show early stages of heart disease. But this evidence did not deter the rating board from denying the claim. Thus, I was forced into the appeal process, which has been ongoing for nearly two years.

There are, however, precautions that can be taken to reduce the ineffectiveness of an examination by an examiner with limited medical skills:

- ◆ Take a companion with you if at all possible so that he or she can attest in a sworn statement that you were only in the examining room for *x* number of minutes. Your companion can also testify if you were sent to other medical services at the clinic, and, if so, which ones. Require that your companion accompany you to the examining room to support your statement later of whether your claim file was available at the time of the evaluation and if the doctor was knowledgeable of your medical history.
- ◆ Determine the examiner's credentials. For example, ask: "Are you a psychiatrist or psychologist?" Find out if the doctor is board-certified in a specialty and whether he or she is currently licensed in the state where the examination was conducted. After the examination, take the time to write the AMA

national headquarters in Chicago, and obtain a background report on the doctor or doctors who examined you. All this information is necessary if you have to refute the examiner's capability to administer a thorough and contemporaneous examination.

♦ Make a list of your medical problems and describe all the symptoms you are experiencing for each medical condition. If you are on medication, list the drug and dosage of each drug used. If the medication has resulted in side effects that are responsible for other medical problems, record this information and make it known to the examiner.

♦ Give the examiner a copy of the credentials and medical assessment by your own private specialist. I have found that in many cases this will intimidate or influence an examiner of a lesser medical background. When it is the VA policy to use minimally qualified examiners to evaluate complex injuries or diseases, it's important that a veteran is able to counter this breach of faith.

Don't Make Assumptions—The VA Is Not Always Right

If your claim is denied, you should not accept the results of a VA medical evaluation as conclusive and absolute. There is a lot riding on the results of a C&P examination and to assume that the VA administered a thorough and contemporaneous examination is a grave mistake that could deny lawful entitlements and care. Do not assume that the VA examining doctor is an expert in the field related to your disability problems. The services of a recognized private specialist should be obtained to refute the medical findings of any VA physician if benefits are denied. This is the only way to protect your interests.

Chapter 7: What Have We Learned?

1. The entire VA system is undergoing a transformation that is not necessarily in the best interest of veterans. The VA Health Administration is currently engaged in an ambitious program to downsize the VA heathcare system and drastically cut costs.

2. One initiative designed to cut healthcare access for veterans across the board was made part of the Veterans Healthcare Reform Act of 1996. Veterans desiring medical treatment from the VA had to enroll in VA Healthcare Program by October 1998. Now, at the time of enrollment, a veteran will be assigned into one of eight priority groups. This program requires that every veteran who is not rated at least 50% disabled must register annually. The priority group to which a veteran is assigned is not permanent and can be adjusted up or down the priority ladder.

3. With the exception of veterans rated 50% or more, the only treatment available to a veteran who is rated less than 50% will be for the actual condition that is service related. The money that is saved with this policy can be redirected to other political goals of the government, totally unrelated to the needs of the citizenry.

4. Primarily, it is minimally trained examiners who perform VA medical services. Basically it is cheaper than providing the kind of specialist required to properly evaluate a serious injury or complex disease. The VA also uses nonphysician medical personnel to conduct C&P examinations. Even though it is alleged that they work under the supervision of a physician, an examination by one of these caregivers cannot meet the VA standards needed for benefit claims.

5. It is an absolute necessity for a veteran to consult with a private medical specialist before being examined by the VA. Your specialist must be provided with medical records of your condition, VA regulations, and manuals that are applicable to your situation. The specialist assessment of your condition must show a clear diagnosis, the limitations it imposes upon you, and how your condition relates to your contention that it is service incurred. The doctor's closing remarks should contain a statement similar to this: "Based on a review of Mr. Smith's service medical records, my examinations and tests, it is my opinion that this condition did in fact occur while he served in the U.S. Army between 1945 and 1955. Using the standards published in 38 *CFR* Part IV Mr. Smith is 60% disabled."

6. By law, the VA must provide you with an examination if the medical evidence submitted with your claim and service medical records are not sufficient to rate your claim. You cannot afford to sit back and expect the VA to adjudicate your claim wisely. To be successful you must know exactly what the VA must do when you are examined. Remember 38 *CFR*, part IV and "AMIE PTSD Protocol Examination" are the tools the VA examiner must work with when he or she evaluates your condition. Know what the examiner should check and if he or she doesn't follow the manual, ask why.

7. Make certain when you are examined that you ask the examiner about his or her credentials and, *most important, whether he or she read and reviewed your claim file prior to the examination.* Don't let the doctor ignore the question; get an answer. Failure to do so is a not only a violation of VA policy but also a violation of federal law. Make this fact known to the examiner even if you are rebuked because of your question. You cannot afford to be passive in these matters. As soon as the examination has been concluded, go out into the waiting room and record everything you remember that was discussed and checked. Record the total time you were with the examiner. If you don't, it may take you three to five years to recover lost ground.

Notes

1. These stories have been pulled from various newspapers, including the St. Petersburg Times, Tampa Tribune, New York Times, Los Angeles Times, and Chicago Tribune.
2. The headlines quoted are from the St. Petersburg Times, St. Petersburg, Florida between April of 1997 and November 1997.
3. U.S. Code 38, chap. 74, §7401–10, 1991.
4. VA manual M21-1, part VI, change 38, dated August 30, 1995.
5. *Irby v. Brown*, 6 F. 12 (Vet. App. 1994).
6. *Sklar v. Brown*, 5 F. 140 (Vet. App. 1993). In *Sklar v. Brown*, the court held that if there is a diagnosis by a specialist and the only evidence against the veteran claim is a contrary opinion by a nonspecialist, then the findings of the nonspecialist should carry little weight.
7. Clinician's Guide (Washington, DC: VA Health Administration, March 2002), http://www.warms.vba.va.gov/admin21/guide/cliniciansguide.doc, 5–21.
8. See *Dusek v. Derwinski*, 2 F. 519 (Vet. App. 1992). In this case, the court ruled that the VA properly denied the veteran's increased benefits because he failed to report for an evaluation examination and failed to provide a good cause for his action. The court noted, "The duty to assist is not always a one-way street."
9. See *Addison v. Brown*, 6 F. 405 (Vet. App. 1994). The court ruled that the VA failed in its duty to assist by relying on an examination that was performed during an inactive stage, that is, when Addison's condition was in remission. The case was remanded and returned to the BVA with instructions to examine the veteran when his condition was active.

8 | TOTAL DISABILITY BASED ON INDIVIDUAL UNEMPLOYABILITY

It is a national commitment to provide every veteran who suffered a service-related disability with compensation to offset the loss of earning capacity owing to the injury or disease. Within this pledge is a special provision whereby a disabled veteran who is unemployable owing to a disability will be compensated at a rate of 100% even if his or her disability is not totally disabling (100%).

The controlling regulations for this provision are 38 *CFR* §3.340(a)(2) and 38 *CFR* §4.16. In addition, the code regulations are backed by numerous court decisions clarifying the intent of Congress. If a veteran is unemployable, this special benefit should be one of the easiest to establish. Unfortunately, it is one of the hardest claims to establish and it is also one of the easiest benefits for the VA to terminate.

In the early 1980s there were more than 100,000 veterans in receipt of Total Disability based on Individual Unemployability (TDIU) benefits. Thus began a movement within the VA to limit entitlement for this benefit. When the Republicans moved into the White House in 1981, President Reagan and his administration moved to cut the cost of social programs. One of the biggest budget gobblers was the Veterans Administration with its compensation and healthcare programs. Thanks to Reagan's efforts to divert funds from the VA and other agencies to his missile projects, by the early 1990s, the number of veterans in receipt of TDIU was reduced to a little more than 60,000 nationwide.

The reduction process was quite simple to initiate. First, the VA ordered a series of reevaluation examinations for veterans in receipt of TDIU. Many veterans were notified that the results of their examination showed their disabilities had improved and they could return to the workplace. Next, the central office in Washington, DC, took over approval for TDIU claims and instructed local RO adjudicators to disregard some well-grounded claims for TDIU benefits.

This policy changed the way the VA handled claims for TDIU and violated the provisions of 38 U.S.C. §7722 (Outreach Services) and 38 *CFR* §3.103(a) (Procedural Due Process and Appellate Rights). *Veterans Advocate* reported that 200 veterans in receipt of TDIU benefits were terminated in November 1992 while the central office approved only five veterans for the benefits.[1] These numbers demonstrate just how clever and ruthless an administration can be when they want to cut benefits.

In 2006 the VA made another attempt to chop billions from its budget. The agency announced that it intended to review 72,000 compensation beneficiaries, rated between 70% and 100%, who could conceivably be overrated for PTSD. VA's data shows that 72,000 was exactly the number of veterans who were rated 70% to 100% in that year. Public and congressional uproar in response to the announcement convinced VA to reconsider. The agency subsequently claimed that its announcement had been misinterpreted and that claims examiners were simply going to review the records for minor administrative errors.

TDIU Issues and the Court

When the U.S. Court of Appeals for Veterans Claims started hearing TDIU cases, it found the adjudication process to be out of line with the laws and regulations governing TDIU issues. The *Veterans Advocate* reported that when the court began deciding TDIU cases, many mistakes and improprieties were found. Some Regional Offices had created secret rules—questionable directives that could possibly be illegal. In addition, basic rules were misinterpreted by rating boards and authorization specialists, and expert medical and vocational opinions were treated as statements of speculation. ROs were not requesting expert vocational opinions prior to deciding cases and, when professional opinions were provided by the claimant attesting to the inability to be gainfully employed, rating boards were ignoring the value of the evidence and were not giving it the same weight as symptoms noted on a C&P examination. Adjudicators also refused to discuss in detail the reasons why claimants were considered to be employable.

Even with decisions of the court defining the intent of the law in TDIU cases, ROs continued to deny claims based on former standards. It seemed too many local ROs continued to do business as usual regardless of what the court instructed adjudication personnel on how to decide a TDIU claim. Two cases decided by two different panels of judges provide excellent examples of the VA doing business as usual. Chief Judge Nebeker declared *Beaty v. Brown* and *James v. Brown* "nearly identical" when writing for the court in *James v. Brown*.[2] He wrote, "This case presents a situation nearly identical to that in *Beaty* in which all the evidence supports the veteran's claim for a TDIU rating. We hold that that the Board's [BVA] decision to the contrary does not have a plausible basis. Accordingly, the Board's decision is REVERSED and the matter REMANDED." The court has rendered numerous TDIU decisions since 1991.

That court decision was published in 1991 and Sgt. David Raz still is fighting the same prejudices that plagued his predecessors. This is why it necessary to know what the regulations are when a VA claims specialist decides a TDIU claim.

The Most Common Reasons TDIU Claims Are Denied

MEDICAL PROBLEMS UNRELATED TO SERVICE
Benefits are often denied for TDIU when the veteran has non-service-related medical problems in addition to service-connected disabilities. The VA will not make a determination based solely on the service-connected medical conditions. Claims examiners contend that the non-service-connected medical problem is a major factor in causing the veteran to be unemployable. If you are denied benefits on these grounds you should reopen your claim and argue that a determination can only be made on the service-related disabilities. Non-service-connected disabilities are irrelevant.

WORKFORCE ATTRITION
The VA denied many claims because the veteran dropped out of the workforce because of a non-service-connected condition or because of age. Again, this is totally irrelevant. The VA can evaluate only the effects of the service-connected condition as it relates to employability. Do your records show the service-connected medical problem can stand alone as a cause of individual unemployability? If so, then you need to reopen your claim and argue that the only relevant issue is your service-connected condition.

OPINION, NOT EVIDENCE
Local rating boards have rebutted unemployability assessments provided by the veteran's own professional vocational evaluators with their own unsubstantiated opinions. One of the first cases involving TDIU before the court was *Colvin v. Derwinski* in which the court ruled that when all the evidence in the record is in favor of the veteran's claim, the VA cannot deny the claim based on opinion instead of on positive evidence to disprove the claim.[3] If your claim was denied on this basis, reopen your claim citing *Colvin v. Derwinski* and 38 *CFR* §3.105(a).

INFORMAL AND FORMAL CLAIMS ACKNOWLEDGMENT
Another error made by the VA in handling TDIU claims is when the VA ignores the original request for this benefit. If you ever served notice to the VA, formally or informally, that you were unable to be gainfully employed because of your service-connected condition, and if the VA did not rate your request at that time, then the claim is still pending.

A formal application is the submission of a completed VA Form 21-8940 (Veteran's Application for Increased Compensation Based on Unemployability). An informal claim is any form of written notice to the VA that states you were unable to work because of your service-connected condition. When the VA receives an informal request for benefits, adjudicators are required to send you the proper form to use to apply for that benefit. Failure to do so is a major error.

RECLASSIFICATION BY CROSS TRAINING

If your records show that you are in receipt of Social Security Disability (SSD) benefits for the same disabilities for which you are service-connected and your doctor states you are not capable of working in your field of employment because of your service-connected condition, you may still be entitled to vocational rehabilitation benefits—which would allow the VA to remove you from the 100% TDIU rating group. VA claims examiners will require an evaluation by a rehabilitation vocational counselor to determine if you are a candidate for possible cross training into another field. You will be required to provide a history of your education and work experiences. If you were previously denied vocational rehabilitation training, you should file a claim to reopen your claim based on new and material evidence.

PSYCHIATRIC DISORDERS RESTRICTIONS

Another group of veterans (other than the thousands of veterans rated less than 70% who are consistently denied TDIU benefits) is those who are consistently denied a 100% disability rating owing to unemployability—because they are disabled by psychiatric disorders and unable to be gainfully employed. Psychiatric disorders as identified in 38 *CFR* §4.125 are psychotic disorders, psychoneurotic disorders, organic mental disorders, and post-traumatic stress disorder. The schedule rating for each of these categories is found in 38 *CFR* §4.132.

If you are a veteran with psychiatric disabilities and you were denied benefits for TDIU, you may have strong grounds to reopen your claim under the provisions of 38 *CFR* §3.105(a) and 38 *CFR* §4.16(b) including decisions by the court in *Murincsak v. Derwinski* and *Gleicher v. Derwinski*.[4] These provisions legally removed the former guideline that restricted interpretation of psychiatric disability. You can reopen your claim based on a CUE (clear and unmistakable error), even after a decision becomes final. Mind you, this method of challenging the VA is not a walk in the park. The court's decisions on CUE cases have been extremely conservative, possibly because if you prevail, the VA must go back to day one when settling the claim resulting in a huge settlement.

Basic Eligibility for TDIU Benefits

The governing regulations for TDIU benefits are 38 *CFR* §3.340(a)(2) and 38 *CFR* §4.16(a)(b). A total disability rating is based on the premise that there is impairment of mind or body that is sufficient to render it impossible for the average person to follow a substantially gainful occupation. In accordance with 38 *CFR* §3.340(a)(2), entitlement to a total disability rating can be established even when the scheduler rating for the condition or conditions is less than 100% disabling.

In 38 *CFR* §4.16(a), the eligibility requirements necessary to receive TDIU benefits when rated less than 100% disabled are spelled out. Subparagraph (a) establishes where the scheduler rating is less than total (less than 100%), but *in the judgment of the rating board member*, you are unable to maintain a substantially gainful occupation, a total disability rating may be assigned. However, to qualify under subparagraph (a) you must have one disability rated at least 60% disabling or have two or more disabilities of which one disability is rated at least 40% and the combined ratings of all disabilities equals 70%.

Adjudicators are told that marginal employment shall not be considered substantially gainful employment. VA policy defines marginal income as annual earned income that does not exceed the poverty threshold for one person.

Subparagraph (b) addresses the needs of a veteran who is rated less than 60% for one disability or the combined disability rating for two or more disabilities is less 70%. It was established to ensure that a veteran unable to qualify for benefits under 38 *CFR* § 3.340(a)(2) or 38 *CFR* §4.16(a) would be considered entitled to total disability benefits if unable to be gainfully employed because of the service-connected disability.

The regulation reads, in part:

> It is the established policy of the Department of Veterans Affairs that all veterans who are unable to secure and follow a substantially gainful occupation by reason of service-connected disabilities *shall be rated totally disabled.* Therefore, *rating boards should submit* to the Director, Compensation and Pension Service, for extra-scheduler consideration on all cases of veterans who are unemployable by reason of service-connected disabilities, but who fail to meet the percentage standards set forth in paragraph (a) of the section. (Italics added.)

The reduction of veterans on the roll or being approved for TDIU benefits stems from several factors. First, 38 *CFR* §4.16(a) grants rating boards considerable leeway in deciding whether the claimant is capable of obtaining and maintaining gainful employment. Allied to this factor of personal judgment, rating board members are not specially trained to equate the medical limitations of the claimant disability to the ability to be gainfully employed.

The court has rendered many decisions addressing the issue of TDIU. In *Gleicher v. Derwinski*, the court held that the VA improperly denied a TDIU claim because it based its denial of benefits on its own unsubstantiated vocational opinion. If TDIU benefits were denied when there was sufficient evidence you were not capable of being gainfully employed and the VA examiners had no evidence to refute your claim other than their personal judgment, you should reopen your claim based on a clear and unmistakable error.

Another reason many veterans experience so much difficulty in gaining approved for TDIU benefits is because ROs seldom follow the intent of the regulation. The veteran is told the requirements set forth in 38 *CFR* §4.18(a) have not been met, therefore the claim is denied. The denial letter cites the percent of disability required to be eligible for TDIU benefits. The veteran is not told TDIU benefits are possible if the service-connected condition, regardless of the rating, is responsible for his or her inability to be gainfully employed. For example, if you are unemployable owing to a psychological disability rated less than 70%, file a claim to reopen your case based on a clear and unmistakable error (38 *CFR* §3.105(a.) The basis of the reopened claim would be that the RO of original jurisdiction failed to comply with the provisions of 38 *CFR* §4.16(b) and forward your claim on to the central office in Washington, DC.

Few veterans and service officers know what the regulations mandate. For example, when initiating a claim, most claimants do not provide the type of evidence that establishes the service-connected condition as responsible for causing the inability to be gainfully employed. Veterans and many advocates do not know that VA doctors, when performing a C&P examination, are to state in their evaluation if the service-connected condition is responsible for the individual's unemployability. The rating board members know this statement should be part of the evaluation report. However, its absence is ignored and so is the provision of 38 *CFR* §4.2 (Interpretation of Examination Reports) that directs a rating board to return the examination to the medical center as being inadequate for evaluation purposes.

The only saving grace is that now the BVA is examining each appeal under guidelines provided by the many court decisions. Unfortunately, the veteran must still wait several years to be granted TDIU benefits while the appeal makes its way through the process.

Gleicher v. Derwinski also addressed what the VA was required to do when a veteran with a scheduler rating of 70% was unemployable solely because of his psychological problem. The VA contention was a veteran with only a service-connected psychological disability was not entitled to TDIU benefits.

Writing for the court, Judge Ronald M. Holdaway held that, "A veteran with a 70% disability rating is entitled to an 'extra scheduler' total disability rating if he is unable to secure or follow a substantially gainful occupation as a result of the disability." The court further stated that in this case "the BVA failed to consider the 1988 VA psychiatric examination report and the 1988 VA social and industrial survey, both of which concluded that the appellant was incapable of securing or maintaining employment." There was no evidence of record to the contrary to rebut the appellant's claim.

Proving a Claim for TDIU Benefits

Always remember that you, the claimant, has the burden to prove your claim. Technically, if your evidence establishes a well-grounded basis for the claim, the VA is required to assist you in fully developing the claim before it is decided. In one of the earliest cases decided before the court, *Colvin v. Derwinski,* the court spelled out the specifics of the VA's duty toward the claimant.[5]

The court ruled that the VA's duty was: (1) to obtain the evidence, (2) to consider the evidence, (3) to evaluate the claim, and (4) to explain, if the claim is denied, how examiners arrived at that decision in light of expert medical and vocational opinions from professional witnesses. They must tell you exactly how they justified the denial of benefits. Regional offices continue to this day to deny claims in spite of the ruling in this case and others like it. For this reason alone, *you have to depend only on yourself to put together a winning claim.* Don't make the mistake of thinking that VA personnel will do all the digging and searching for evidence that will grant you the benefits claimed.

Proving up your claim is not a difficult task if you understand exactly what kind of evidence is needed to get the job done. You must know the rules the VA is supposed to follow. TDIU claims must prove that your service-connected disability alone is responsible for your inability to be gainfully employed. There are five sources of evidence to include in a well-documented TDIU claim: expert medical proof, vocational proof, a sworn statement by the veteran, sworn statements from former or prospective employers who rejected your application for employment because of your service-connected disability, and a copy of your Social Security award letter which confirms Social Security disability benefits based on your service-connected medical problems. Taking the time to put together a well-documented claim will avoid the pitfalls most veterans face.

MEDICAL EVIDENCE
First, obtain an expert medical assessment from your own physician. The doctor must explain in writing exactly how your service-connected disability affects your ability to be gainfully employed. Should you have an additional disability that is not service-connected, explain to the doctor that the report must address only your service-connected condition. However, if your doctor could make a statement to the effect that your non-service-connected conditions would not or could not be the cause of your unemployability, have the doctor do so. Do not let the doctor lump all your disabilities

together and give a generalized report. The danger here is, if the report offers the slightest doubt that your service-connected condition is not responsible for your un-employability, the VA will deny the claim.

If you are being treated solely by a VA medical service for your service-connected condition, it is doubtful that the VA physician will put together the kind of letter you need. He or she will tell you verbally that because of your service-connected condition, you can't work, but the physician is often extremely reluctant to put it in writing. In my own experience with VA doctors, I was never successful when trying to obtain the type of letter necessary to prove unemployability on behalf of my clients.

One last thought on medical evidence: You cannot afford *not* to have an assessment by a specialist in the field related to your disability. When you see the specialist, state up front that you want an evaluation concerning your service-connected condition and its effects on your ability to be gainfully employed. The doctor must understand that this report *must* be in writing. If the doctor resists providing a written report, don't invest anymore of your money or time. Find someone who will meet your needs. Remember that you have a lot riding on this claim: more than $2,000 per month, for life. The cost of a first-rate medical work-up should not deter you from obtaining the examination.

Once you have located a specialist, your next job is to explain what you need in order to qualify for TDIU benefits. You must provide the following tools for the specialist and your physician:

♦   copy of your complete VA claim file;
♦   copies of Social Security Disability (SSD) decisions and the evidence used to grant SSD benefits (detailed copies of Social Security records can be obtained under the Freedom of Information Act via your congressional representative's office);
♦   copies of all medical evidence from private physicians;
♦   copies of any sworn statements from former employers that terminated your employment because of your disability;
♦   copy of any special educational training you may have completed;
♦   copies of high school, college, or technical school transcripts;
♦   copy of the pertinent paragraphs from 38 *CFR*, part 3 and 4 that apply to your disability.

VOCATIONAL EVIDENCE

The second most important step in supporting your claim is an evaluation by a professional counselor. Developing an unimpeachable source of evidence requires the claimant to be dogged in the search for a professional vocational counselor. The counselor's credentials are critical to your case.

A professional vocational counselor's educational background will range from a bachelor's degree to a doctoral degree (PhD) in vocational counseling. If you have a choice, select an individual with a PhD in vocational counseling. Remember, you are going to battle against any negative conclusions drawn by a rating board member who has had no special training to qualify as a vocational expert. If you are forced to go to appeal, the higher the credentials of your vocational counselor, the greater your chances are of having the decision reversed on appeal.

If you have no idea where to start your search for a vocational specialist, begin with the closest legal service that helps indigent individuals in civil cases. Your local bar association should have the contact information for this legal service. These services do a great deal of litigating on behalf of clients who have been denied Social Security disability benefits. They will be able to put you in touch with a vocational specialist who is experienced in dealing with the government. The upside of hiring a specialist with this kind of experience is that they know how to prepare a written evaluation that has all the right buzz words, and they understand the bureaucratic obstacles you are trying to hurdle over.

It's important that the vocational specialist understand what the VA means by "marginal employment," as opposed to "substantial, gainful employment." This meaning is spelled out in 38 *CFR* §4.16(a), which explains the basic rules for granting TDIU benefits to a veteran with a disability rating less than 70%. Make sure the vocational specialist is aware that age and non-service-connected disabilities are irrelevant in the decision-making process. The only issue that the vocational specialist must address is whether your service-connected disabilities alone would prevent you from obtaining gainful employment.

CLAIMANT'S SWORN STATEMENT AS EVIDENCE
Preparing a sworn statement is not as complicated as it sounds. The statement will include your name, VA claim number or Social Security number, current address, and a sentence to the effect that the statement is true and correct to the best of your knowledge. It should be signed before a notary public. This will ensure that your statement is in compliance with 38 *CFR* §3.200(b). The format of the letter should be a series of direct statements of fact such as is seen in figure 8.1. For another good example, refer back to chapter 3 for Sergeant Raz's sworn statement.

Fig. 8.1

Sworn Declaration of John Doe

1. I live at 782 Lincoln Road, Boonville, Texas, 11111.

2. I have not worked since January 5, 1996.

3. I am service connected for post-traumatic stress disorder at 50%.

4. Before my employment was terminated, I worked at Cooper & Sons, where I worked in the shipping department lifting packages up to 50 pounds. When I could no longer tolerate constant criticism from the supervisor, I exploded with anger, which resulted in being fired. I had no other skills or education that might let me train for another job within the company.

5. I have tried to obtain other jobs, but when it was learned that I suffered from PTSD and was taking prescribed controlled substances, my applications were rejected. I was awarded Social Security Disability benefits because I was unemployable. Each day I have to take six different medications for my heart condition and PTSD.

6. I declare under the penalty of perjury that the above statement is true and correct to the best of my knowledge.

Signature of John Doe

Notary's seal and certification

LAY STATEMENT IN SUPPORT OF YOUR CLAIM

A lay statement is support for your claim from anyone who can provide factual information as to how your service-connected disability affects your ability to work. Lay evidence can be from your spouse, family members, close friends, former employers, or prospective employers who declined to hire you because of your service-connected disability. The statement should be sworn if possible; a sworn statement is preferable and in compliance with 38 *CFR* §3.200(b).

The VA has often dismissively referred to this type of statement as a "buddy letter," but it should be considered valid evidence. Until Congress gave every veteran a source (Court of Appeals for Veterans Claims) to challenge BVA decisions when disputed, lay evidence was seldom given any evidentiary weight. However, rating boards cannot ignore this evidence or fail to give it proper evidentiary weight. Two cases decided early on by the court, *Colvin v. Derwinski* and *Cartright v. Derwinski,* held that lay evidence, in and of itself, might warrant service connection.[6]

Both 38 *CFR* §3.200(b) and 38 *CFR* §3.307(b) dictate how the VA will treat lay evidence in determining the granting of specific benefits sought. First, 38 *CFR* §3.200(b) instructs: "All written testimony submitted by the claimant or in his or her behalf for the purpose of establishing a claim for service connection will be certified or under oath or affirmation." In referring to the adjudication process of deciding a claim, 38 *CFR* §3.307(b) states, in part, "The factual basis may be established by medical evidence, competent lay evidence or both."

As previously discussed, a lay statement under oath should be simple and direct, stating only facts, not opinions or conjecture. The same basic format that was outlined for a veteran's statement (fig. 8.1) can be adapted for use by anyone.

SOCIAL SECURITY DISABILITY EVIDENCE

A veteran that has been granted Social Security Disability benefits for the same condition that is service connected can thank the court for giving them a major leg up toward being granted TDIU benefits. The first four cases concerning the impact of SSD benefits (*Collier v. Derwinski, Murincsak v. Derwinski, Brown v. Derwinski,* and *Shoemaker v. Derwinski*) clearly defined what the VA must consider and do when a veteran is in receipt of SSD benefits for the same reason the veteran is receiving compensation benefits.[7] Despite these case rulings, the VA continued to dismiss the importance of a claimant in receipt of SSD benefits and these subsequent cases also dealt with this issue: *Masors v. Derwinski, Clarkson v. Brown, Beaty v. Brown,* and *James v. Brown.*[8]

These are the basic ground rules the VA must follow when adjudicating a claim where the veteran is in receipt of SSD benefits for the same condition or conditions that granted him or her VA compensation benefits:

- ◆ A SSD claim cannot be ignored and, to the extent its conclusions are not accepted, the reasons should be clearly stated.
- ◆ A determination by the Social Security Administration (SSA) that a claimant is entitled to disability benefits is relevant to a VA determination of the severity of claimant's disability. Further, the court held that SSA disability ratings are not outdated for the purpose of making a determination, since SSA continuously reviews eligibility for disability benefits.
- ◆ When reviewing a well-grounded claim for TDIU benefits where the claimant is recognized as unemployable by SSA, the VA must consider entitlement under 38 *CFR* §4.16(b), even if the condition is rated less than those standards required by 38 *CFR* §4.16(a). In theory if you had a 10% disability, and Social Security determined you were unemployable, the VA would be required to grant the benefit or prove your employability, both vocationally and medically.

- ◆ The VA must obtain and review the claimant's Social Security records when put on notice that he or she is receiving SSD benefits.
- ◆ The VA cannot justify the denial of TDIU benefits with the argument that SSA disability determinations are based on a different set of standards. If the VA rejects the findings of your SSA disability determination, claims examiners must state in detail exactly what evidence they have that is superior to the SSA decision granting benefits and why the SSA determination is not relevant in your case.

VA adjudicators lack the initiative to request SSA records and associated medical records so this point is still a losing battle for most veterans. In spite of all the cases decided by the CAVC on this issue and all the remands by the BVA, the ROs are still not doing their job.

Let me give you example of a BVA case that illustrates this issue perfectly. Appeals from 1994 and 1995 are available on the BVA website. A search under the heading TDIU brought up more than thirty decisions where TDIU was the issue on the appeal. BVA case number 950971, docket number 93-15-575 dealt with a claim for TDIU benefits that had to be remanded back to the RO. The RO failed to obtain the SSA records when the record showed the veteran had made it known to the RO that he was getting SSD for the same reasons he was receiving service-connected benefits. The case goes back to 1993, when the case appeared before the BVA. The BVA remanded the case back to the RO in 1995. Another six months to a year are allowed before the case is recycled and decided. If the RO still denies TDIU, it will be another couple of years before it is reviewed once again by the BVA. This is a very long time for a veteran to live with a greatly reduced income. There is no justifiable excuse for the RO to fail in its duty to assist by not obtaining those records the moment the claims examiner was advised SSA records would be relevant to this claim.

If you were denied TDIU benefits in the past because the VA did not consider the records and decision of SSA, you should reopen your claim based on a clear and unmistakable error under 38 *CFR* §3.105(a.) If you were told that you did not qualify for TDIU benefits because your service-connected disabilities did not qualify under 38 *CFR* §4.16(a), you'll want to reopen your claim if you were in receipt of SSA benefits for the same reasons you were granted service connection.

Applying for TDIU Benefits

AN INFORMAL CLAIM
The first step in applying for TDIU benefits is to file an informal claim. This action will:

- protect your entitlement date;
- give you one year from the date the VA furnishes the formal application form (VA form 21-8490) to submit your claim for consideration;
- enable you to get a complete copy of your VA claim file.

Arrange for a medical and vocational assessment to document your claim that you are too disabled to work. Obtain sworn lay statements, including sworn testimony by you, describing how your service-connected condition has prevented you from maintaining gainful employment. Obtain copies of all your Social Security Disability records to support your claim that you are unemployable. Apply for SSD benefits, if you haven't already done so, and have your claim for SSA benefits decided.

An informal claim is a written notification to the VA that you *intend* to file a claim for Total Disability based on Individual Unemployability. The statement should be short and to the point. For example:

Please accept this action as my informal notice to apply for Total Disability Benefits Due to Individual Unemployability. My service-connected PTSD condition has made it impossible for me to continue to be gainfully employed. A formal application will be submitted once I receive the formal application and I have obtained the medical and vocational evidence necessary to grant TDIU.

I also request that I be furnished a complete copy of my VA claim file at the earliest possible date so it will be available to my doctors and vocational counselors for review along with an official application form.

FORMAL APPLICATION FOR TDIU BENEFITS

Unless you have a completely documented claim, ready to be filed, do not file an original application for TDIU benefits initially. *It's a major tactical error to go to the VA with a claim that is not well documented and supported by solid evidence.* You should take charge of putting together your own claim. If you err at this point, it's all over but for the cussing. Your only recourse will be to appeal the denial of benefits. Two to three years later, your case will be reviewed by the BVA and the only issue on appeal is, was your claim a well-grounded claim? If claims reviewers affirm the decision of the RO, your last recourse is the Court of Appeals for Veterans Claims. Let's assume that nearly five years have gone by and the court reverses the BVA. Now we go all the way back to square one and determine if your service-connected condition will entitle you to TDUI benefits based on the evidence in the record at the time of application.

To claim TDIU benefits you must initiate a claim action on VA Form 21-8940 and submit it to the RO that services the area where you live. Unless you have obtained all of the evidence previously discussed, *do not* call the VA on their toll free number (1-800-827-1000) and request the official application form. Make them respond to your written informal claim notice and provide a formal application by mail.

If the VA has not provided you with the application (as they are required to do by law), send them a certified letter telling them this is your second request for a TDIU application. Attach a copy of the first request putting them on notice that you are applying for TDIU benefits. *Don't do business with the VA by telephone*; any transactions you conclude with them cannot be verified or proven. It's your word against theirs, and you won't get the benefit of doubt. Just remember what the gold miners in California had to deal with when they turned over their laundry to the Chinese shop owners and then tried to claim their laundry without a ticket: "No tickee, no laundry, so sorry." Without proof, you're in the same boat as the miners of 1849.

The application form is fairly straightforward and, after requesting some basic information about the claimant, is divided into four specialized sections: Section I, Disability and Medical Treatment; Section II, Employment History; Section III, Schooling and Training; and Section IV, Authorizations, Certifications and Signature releases.

OMB Approved No. 2900-0404
Respondent Burden: 45 minutes

Department of Veterans Affairs	**VETERAN'S APPLICATION FOR INCREASED COMPENSATION BASED ON UNEMPLOYABILITY**

NOTE: This is a claim for compensation benefits based on unemployability. When you complete this form you are claiming total disability because of a service-connected disability(ies) which has/have prevented you from securing or following any substantially gainful occupation. Answer all questions fully and accurately.

Social Security Benefits: Individuals who have a disability and meet medical criteria may qualify for Social Security or Supplemental Security Income disability benefits. If you would like more information about Social Security benefits, contact your nearest Social Security Administration (SSA) office. You can locate the address of the nearest SSA office in your telephone book blue pages under "United States Government, Social Security Administration" or call 1-800-772-1213 (Hearing Impaired TDD line 1-800-325-0778). You may also contact SSA by Internet at http://www.ssa.gov/.

1. VA FILE NUMBER	2. VETERAN'S SOCIAL SECURITY NUMBER	3. DATE OF BIRTH

4. NAME OF VETERAN *(First, Middle, Last) (Type or Print)*	5. ADDRESS OF CLAIMANT *(No. and street or rural route, city or P.O., State and ZIP Code)*

SECTION I - DISABILITY AND MEDICAL TREATMENT

6. WHAT SERVICE-CONNECTED DISABILITY PREVENTS YOU FROM SECURING OR FOLLOWING ANY SUBSTANTIALLY GAINFUL OCCUPATION?	7. HAVE YOU BEEN UNDER A DOCTOR'S CARE AND/OR HOSPITALIZED WITHIN THE PAST 12 MONTHS?	8. DATE(S) OF TREATMENT BY DOCTOR(S)

9. NAME AND ADDRESS OF DOCTOR(S)	10. NAME AND ADDRESS OF HOSPITAL	11. DATE(S) OF HOSPITALIZATION

SECTION II - EMPLOYMENT STATEMENT

12. DATE YOUR DISABILITY AFFECTED FULL-TIME EMPLOYMENT	13. DATE YOU LAST WORKED FULL-TIME	14. DATE YOU BECAME TOO DISABLED TO WORK

15A. WHAT IS THE MOST YOU EVER EARNED IN ONE YEAR? $	15B. WHAT YEAR?	15C. OCCUPATION DURING THAT YEAR

16. LIST ALL YOUR EMPLOYMENT INCLUDING SELF-EMPLOYMENT FOR THE LAST FIVE YEARS YOU WORKED

A. NAME AND ADDRESS OF EMPLOYER	B. TYPE OF WORK	C. HOURS PER WEEK	D. DATES OF EMPLOYMENT FROM	D. DATES OF EMPLOYMENT TO	E. TIME LOST FROM ILLNESS	F. HIGHEST GROSS EARNINGS PER MONTH

G. INDICATE YOUR TOTAL EARNED INCOME FOR THE PAST 12 MONTHS $	H. IF PRESENTLY EMPLOYED, INDICATE YOUR CURRENT MONTHLY EARNED INCOME $

17. DID YOU LEAVE YOUR LAST JOB/SELF-EMPLOYMENT BECAUSE OF YOUR DISABILITY? ☐ YES ☐ NO *(If "Yes," give the facts in Item 24)*	18. DO YOU RECEIVE/EXPECT TO RECEIVE DISABILITY RETIREMENT BENEFITS? ☐ YES ☐ NO	19. DO YOU RECEIVE/EXPECT TO RECEIVE WORKERS COMPENSATION BENEFITS? ☐ YES ☐ NO

20. HAVE YOU TRIED TO OBTAIN EMPLOYMENT SINCE YOU BECAME TOO DISABLED TO WORK?
☐ YES ☐ NO *(If "Yes," complete Items A, B, and C)*

A. NAME AND ADDRESS OF EMPLOYER	B. TYPE OF WORK	C. DATE APPLIED

VA FORM OCT 2004 **21-8940**

SUPERSEDES VA FORM 21-8940, MAR 2000, WHICH WILL NOT BE USED.

SECTION III - SCHOOLING AND OTHER TRAINING

21. EDUCATION *(Circle highest year completed)*

GRADE SCHOOL 1 2 3 4 5 6 7 8   HIGH SCHOOL 1 2 3 4   COLLEGE 1 2 3 4

22A. DID YOU HAVE ANY OTHER EDUCATION AND TRAINING BEFORE YOU WERE TOO DISABLED TO WORK?

☐ YES ☐ NO   *(If "Yes," complete Items 22B and 22C)*

22B. TYPE OF EDUCATION OR TRAINING	22C. DATES OF TRAINING	
	BEGINNING	COMPLETION

23A. HAVE YOU HAD ANY EDUCATION AND TRAINING SINCE YOU BECAME TOO DISABLED TO WORK?

☐ YES ☐ NO   *(If "Yes," complete Items 23B and 23C)*

23B. TYPE OF EDUCATION OR TRAINING	23C. DATES OF TRAINING	
	BEGINNING	COMPLETION

24. REMARKS

SECTION IV - AUTHORIZATION, CERTIFICATION, AND SIGNATURE

AUTHORIZATION FOR RELEASE OF INFORMATION: I authorize the person or entity, including but not limited to any organization, service provider, employer, or Government agency, to give the Department of Veterans Affairs any information about me except protected health information, and I waive any privilege which makes the information confidential.

CERTIFICATION OF STATEMENTS: I CERTIFY THAT as a result of my service-connected disabilities, I am unable to secure or follow *any* substantially gainful occupation and that the statements in this application are true and complete to the best of my knowledge and belief. I understand that these statements will be considered in determining my eligibility for VA benefits based on unemployability because of service-connected disability.

I UNDERSTAND THAT IF I AM GRANTED SERVICE-CONNECTED TOTAL DISABILITY BENEFITS BASED ON MY UNEMPLOYABILITY, I MUST IMMEDIATELY INFORM VA IF I RETURN TO WORK. I ALSO UNDERSTAND THAT TOTAL DISABILITY BENEFITS PAID TO ME AFTER I BEGIN WORK MAY BE CONSIDERED AN OVERPAYMENT REQUIRING REPAYMENT TO VA.

25. SIGNATURE OF CLAIMANT	26. DATE SIGNED	27. TELEPHONE NUMBER(S) *(Include Area Code)*	
		A. DAYTIME	B. NIGHTTIME

WITNESS TO SIGNATURE OF CLAIMANT IF MADE BY "X" MARK. NOTE: Signature made by mark must be witnessed by two persons to whom the person making the statement is personally known and the signature and address of such witnesses must be shown below.

28A. SIGNATURE OF WITNESS	28B. ADDRESS OF WITNESS
29A. SIGNATURE OF WITNESS	29B. ADDRESS OF WITNESS

PENALTY: The law provides severe penalties which include fine or imprisonment or both for the willful submission of any statement or evidence of a material fact, knowing it to be false or for the fraudulent acceptance of any payment to which you are not entitled.

PRIVACY ACT NOTICE: VA will not disclose information collected on this form to any source other than what has been authorized under the Privacy Act of 1974 or Title 38, Code of Federal Regulations 1.576 for routine uses (i.e., civil or criminal law enforcement, congressional communications, epidemiological or research studies, the collection of money owed to the United States, litigation in which the United States is a party or has an interest, the administration of VA programs and delivery of VA benefits, verification of identity and status, and personnel administration) as identified in the VA system of records, 58VA21/22, Compensation, Pension, Education and Rehabilitation Records - VA, published in the Federal Register. Your obligation to respond is required to obtain or retain benefits. Giving us your SSN account information is mandatory. Applicants are required to provide their SSN under Title 38, U.S.C. 5101(c)(1). VA will not deny an individual benefits for refusing to provide his or her SSN unless the disclosure of the SSN is required by a Federal Statute of law in effect prior to January 1, 1975, and still in effect. The requested information is considered relevant and necessary to determine maximum benefits provided under the law. The responses you submit are considered confidential (38 U.S.C. 5701). Information submitted is subject to verification through computer matching programs with other agencies.

RESPONDENT BURDEN: We need this information to determine eligibility for individual unemployability (38 U.S.C. 1163). Title 38, United States Code, allows us to ask for this information. We estimate that you will need an average of 45 minutes to review the instructions, find the information, and complete this form. VA cannot conduct or sponsor a collection of information unless a valid OMB control number is displayed. You are not required to respond to a collection of information if this number is not displayed. Valid OMB control numbers can be located on the OMB Internet Page at www.whitehouse.gov/omb/library/OMBINV.html#VA. If desired, you can call 1-800-827-1000 to get information on where to send comments or suggestions about this form.

Basic Identification of Claimant

The first six items on the application are for identification only. It asks for both your Social Security number and VA claim number. If your original claim for benefits dates back to the mid 1970s or later, most likely the VA assigned your Social Security number as your VA claim number. Prior to the changeover, a VA claim number was an eight-digit number preceded by "C," (e.g., C-00-000-000). If you do not know your "C–Number," you can obtain it by contacting the nearest local RO. Its identification system can cross-check your name, date of birth, military serial number, or Social Security number to find out your C-Number.

Section I: Disability and Medical Treatment

Items 7 through 12 require a considerable amount of information to support your claim for TDIU benefits, with very little space provided to do so. The best way to complete the form under these circumstances is to enter into each box, "See attachment for details." When recording the information on the attachment for item 7, for example, write, "Item 7: Lower back injury, gunshot wound to left forearm and right calf; residual damage to liver owing to infectious hepatitis."

Items 9 and 10 should be combined when there is more than one doctor involved. For example: Dr. Robert Smith, 1000 S. Turner Street, Winston, OH, 55441, April 2, 1986, to date; Dr. Elizabeth D. Green, 2230 N. Main Street, Winston, OH, 55442, July 30, 1990, to date; Dr. Harry G. Hart, 315 Harrison Blvd., Winston, OH, 55446, September 3, 1993, to date. You should follow the same format for Items 11 and 12 if you had multiple hospitalizations related to your service-connected disabilities. Make certain that on each attached page you print your name, VA claim number, and Social Security number. You should also note how many pages are attached and what this particular page number is. For example, "Page 1 of 3 pages," "Page 2 of 3 pages," and so on.

Section II: Employment Statement

The dates for Items 13, 14, and 15 could be one date or could reflect three entirely different dates, depending on the circumstances involved. For example, if the claimant was doing physical work and his shoulder, arms, and right leg caused him extreme pain to the extent that he could no longer perform his assigned tasks, this would the be the date his disabilities affected his full-time employment. He may have stayed out of work on sick leave for a month, returned to work, then found he could no longer perform any of his duties. His employer terminated his employment effective the end of the following month because he was using up his accrued vacation time.

Item 17 asks for your employment history for the past five years. Normally this is a one- or two-line entry if you have worked for the same employer for at least seven years before changing jobs.

Items 18 through 21 raise several questions that need to be discussed. Item 18 would normally be checked "no." Item 20 would normally be checked "no." However, if in fact you were in receipt of federal workman's compensation benefits (see 38 *CFR* §3.958) the law prohibits concurrent payments of VA Compensation benefits and Workmen's Compensation benefits after September 13, 1960. The VA requires a detailed explanation in Item 24 as to why your disability forced you to leave your job. The space provided to answer Item 24 is inadequate for a detailed explanation. Note in Item 24, "See attachment, page 2 for explanation of reasons disability caused me to become unemployable."

Section III: Schooling and Other Training

Items 22 through 24 provide the VA with some insight into your potential for employment in another occupation field. Veterans with a college education or other special training are usually considered employable. This is why it's essential that you retain the services of a well-qualified vocational specialist who will weigh all factors of your background before making a determination as to your employability.

I have seen the VA deny TDIU benefits based on the assumption the claimant's college degree made him employable. This one fact rose above the findings of his doctor, who explained why he was unable to be gainfully employed. Remember that these rating specialists do not have any special medical, legal, or vocational training. What they *do* have is the authority to use their own judgment. Your claim has to be well supported by expert evidence or it's going to be years before you see TDIU benefits.

Section IV: Authorization and Certification

The authorization section of VA Form 21-8940 requires that the claimant grant permission for the VA to solicit information from the doctors, surgeons, hospitals, or dentists who have treated you. You are giving claims examiners permission to obtain *any background information* these sources may have. When you sign the application, you are automatically granting them the right to contact anyone to obtain information about you.

The certification portion of Section IV is where you affirm that all statements made are true and correct to the best of your knowledge. Further, it states that you certify that your service-connected disabilities do not permit you to follow *any* substantially gainful occupation. I believe the only reason the VA highlighted the word "any" is to intimidate the claimant. It reminds one of the early days of the Reagan administration when thousands of individuals were taken off the Social Security Disability rolls under the assumption that "everyone can do something." However, the Office of Administrative Law Judges (OALJ) reinstated benefits to these individuals as fast as the cases could be processed. OALJ did not uphold the concept that everybody can be substantially and gainfully employed.

Chapter 8: What Have We Learned?

Congress introduced the Total Disability based on Individual Unemployability (TDIU) benefit program for veterans who were not rated 100% disabled, but who were unable to be gainfully employed because of a service-connected injury, disease, or condition. The program recognized that such veterans should not be deprived of the basic standards of life. It was Congress's intent that the VA should administer this new law under liberal guidelines.

However, this is an entitlement that disabled veterans have been refused more often than any other. The reason is quite simple: it takes a big chunk of money out of the VA budget. During the early 1980s, primarily under the Reagan/Bush administration, more than 40,000 veterans were removed from the TDIU rolls, not because they suddenly became employable, but because they lacked the knowledge and tools to counter the decision. In one decade, the VA reduced its budgetary requirements by $80 million. This amount does not include the savings generated by denying thousands of claims for TDIU benefits between 1980 and 1990.

During this timeframe the VA was acting as its counsel, jury, and, judge for all claims. The Board of Veterans Appeals seldom reversed the rulings of ROs. Only 15% of the cases appearing before the BVA were reversed or remanded. Today, nearly 80% of the appeals being reviewed by the BVA are remanded or reversed.

The shift toward making the ROs do their jobs correctly was not because of a change in policy, training, or a deep commitment to do what was right. The driving force behind this unprecedented turnabout was the decisions of the Court of Appeals for Veterans Claims. The court has been reviewing appeals cases—many of which have dealt with TDIU benefits—since February 1990 and only now is the BVA reviewing appeals with an eye on the intent of Congress.

There are eight court decisions cases cited in this chapter that specifically address the issue of why a veteran in receipt of Social Security Disability (SSD) benefits should not arbitrarily be denied compensation benefits. These benefits will remain some of the most difficult to obtain until Regional Offices apply the intent of the law to the facts of the case and realize that they are not a HMO measuring the amount of black ink on a profit and loss statement.

If you are a veteran who has been denied TDIU benefits or who was removed from the rolls, this is a very important chapter for you. The eligibility requirements are quite broad and uncomplicated. If you are unemployable because of a service-related disability, you are entitled to a special rating of 100%. The key is that you must be unemployable because of your *service-connected disability*. The VA will put considerable effort into abutting your claim, based on the premise that your unemployability can be traced to reasons unrelated to your service-connected disabilities. ROs are notorious for denying TDIU claims based on their own unsubstantiated conclusions.

Notes

1. Ronald Abrams, "Court Decision Exposes Erroneous VA Adjudication of Individual Unemployability Claims," *Veterans Advocate* 4, no.3 (November 1992): 17–24.
2. *Beaty v. Brown*, 6 F. 532 (Vet. App. 1994); and *James v. Brown*, 7 F. 495 (Vet. App. 1995).
3. *Colvin v. Derwinski*, 1 F. 171 (Vet. App. 1991).
4. *Murincsak v. Derwinski*, 2 F. 363 (Vet. App. 1992); and *Gleicher v. Derwinski*, 2 F. 26 (Vet. App. 1991).
5. *Colvin v. Derwinski*, 1 F. 171 (Vet. App. 1991).
6. *Colvin v. Derwinski*, 1 F. 171 (Vet. App. 1991); and *Cartright v. Derwinski*, 2 F. 24 (Vet. App. 1991).
7. *Collier v. Derwinski*, 1 F. 413 (Vet. App. 1991), *Murincsak v. Derwinski*, 2 F. 363 (Vet. App. 1992), *Brown v. Derwinski*, 2 F. 444 (Vet. App. 1992), and *Shoemaker v. Derwinski*, 3 F. 248 (Vet. App. 1992).
8. *Masors v. Derwinski*, 2 F. 181 (Vet. App. 1992), *Clarkson v. Brown*, 4 F. 565 (Vet. App. 1993), *Beaty v. Brown*, 6 F. 532 (Vet. App. 1994), *James v. Brown*, 7 F. 495 (Vet. App. 1995).

Prove Your Case and File Your Claim *or* You Will Be Forced to Defend It on Appeal

Knowing what evidence the VA requires is an absolute must if you expect to submit a winning claim. You cannot win if you

- ◆ cannot protect your interest in the decision-making process because you do not know what the regulations dictate.
- ◆ are unable to submit a well-supported claim that is supported by evidence.
- ◆ do not know how to go about collecting this evidence. You cannot win if you do not know why the VA denies valid claims.
- ◆ assume the VA is an all-knowing agency and that you can rely upon its skills to adjudicate the facts of the case accurately and fairly.

What do the regulations say about your claim before benefits can be granted? To answer that question you need to obtain a copy of the pertinent section of 38 *CFR*, parts III and IV. If you have access to a computer, search the Internet for the information. If you need to make copies of pertinent sections of the regulations, look to the local law library in your county, your VA Regional Office reading room, or a university library designated as a federal depository.

When you are ready, make certain that you know how to put your claim together and the method used in filing. A VA claims examiner will deny your claim if the medical evidence is not persuasive. Organize all your evidence in a logical order and provide a table of exhibits so that you can expect the examiner to rule in your favor. Take no short cuts. Include all required evidence in an orderly manner. Remember that you hold the burden of proving the claim. If you can't do that, for the next two or three years you will argue only one issue: was the evidence sufficient to grant the benefit?

The assembly of your claim and all its supporting evidence must follow a logical path. Each piece of evidence must link to the next and so on, otherwise you put your claim for benefits in harm's way. Identify every piece of paper that is attached to the claim. Number your pages. Mail your claim and documentation by Certified Mail with Return Receipt Requested. If you deliver your claim in person to the VA and you have no proof of exactly what you provided, it could cost you your benefits. Lost documents, forms, statements, and evidence will hurt only you.

You are a veteran. You have the GI Bill of Rights to protect you. Seek out competent advocates to help you through every step and who are knowledgeable about the VA's obligations. Find your evidence, build your case, back up your claim, and follow through until you receive your benefits.

If you need more detailed information regarding how to support your claim, knowing the VA requirements, finding resources, gathering evidence, and successfully filing your claim, please read my previous book, *The Veterans Survival Guide: How to File and Collect on VA Claims*. Also, you may wish to visit these websites:

American Medical Association physician member locator: http://webapps.ama-assn.org/doctorfinder/home.html

Board of Veterans' Appeals (BVA): http://www.va.gov/vbs/bva/

Compensation and Pension (C&P) Examinations: http://www1.va.gov/vhapublications/ViewPublication.asp?pub_ID=1400

C&P Service Clinician's Guide: http://www.warms.vba.va.gov/admin21/guide/cliniciansguide.doc

The Code of Federal Regulations: http://www.gpoaccess.gov/cfr/index.html

Federal Register: http://www.gpoaccess.gov/fr/index.html

InfoSpace: http://www.infospace.com/

National Medical Association (African American) physician locator: http://0081be6.netsolhost.com/index.asp

National Personnel Records Center: http://www.archives.gov/st-louis/military-personnel/

U.S. Army military history: http://www.armyhistory.org/armyhistorical.aspx?pgID=889

U.S. Armed Services Center for Research of Unit Records: http://acronyms.thefreedictionary.com/United+States+Armed+Services+Center+for+Research+of+Unit+Records

U.S. Code: http://www.gpoaccess.gov/uscode/index.html

U.S. Court of Appeals for the Federal Circuit: http://fedcir.gov/

U.S. Court of Appeals for Veterans Claims: http://www.vetapp.uscourts.gov/

U.S. Department of Veterans Affairs, Veterans Benefits Administration: http://www.vba.va.gov/

U.S. National Archives and Records Administration: http://www.gpoaccess.gov/nara/index.html

The Court at Work Protecting PTSD Claims

The U.S. Court of Appeals for the Federal Circuit and the U.S. Court of Appeals for Veterans Claims have addressed many of the issues that have denied veterans PTSD benefits for years. For this chapter, I've selected a cross-section of cases decided by these courts that represent the major reasons why the VA turned down claims.

To give you a sense of how the VA is holding the line on denying service connection for PTSD and substance abuse, here is some startling information: between 1989 and 2004, 819 PTSD cases have been reviewed by the court. The appeals for substance abuse as secondary to PTSD number 57 during this same period. It would take volumes to tell the stories of the nearly 900 PTSD appeals decided by the court. What these numbers don't tell us is how many original, amended, or reopened claims for PTSD or substance abuse were denied by the VA where the veteran did not challenge the decision in the court.

As I worked on this chapter, I became curious how many claims have been filed for PTSD since the very beginning of the Vietnam War through 2003. I wanted to know how many were approved, how many were denied, and, if granted, what percentage of disability was granted. To my knowledge this information has never been made public. In order to reduce the time I would have to wait for this information under the Freedom of Information Act, I asked my congressional representative to forward my request to the VA. Their answer to me was "We do not collect or correlate this type information." Yeah, right! See figure 9.1 to read how their letter explains it to me.

Fig. 9.1

DEPARTMENT OF VETERANS AFFAIRS
Veterans Benefits Administration
Washington, D.C. 20420

Nov. 10, 2004

The Honorable Michael Bilirakis
Member, U. S. House of Representatives
35111 U- S. Highway 19 North, Suite 301
Palm Harbor, FL 34684

Dear Congressman Bilirakis;

I am pleased to respond to your letter concerning your constituent, Mr. John D. Roche, and his request, under provisions of the Freedom of Information Act (FOIA), for statistics on the number of veterans who filed claims for Post Traumatic Stress Disorder (PTSD) from 1961 to 2003. Mr. Roche would also like the information broken down by how many claims were approved, with their associated percentage rating, or denied.

The Department of Veterans Affairs (VA) did not recognize or designate PTSD as a separate disability diagnostic code (9411) until 1980- Therefore, we are unable to furnish the specific information requested. In addition, we do not maintain a report on the number of PTSD claims denied. However, enclosed for Mr. Roche's consideration, is a record of the number of veterans rated for PTSD, with associated percentage disability, from 1986 to 2004.

I hope this information is of assistance to you in responding to Mr. Roche.

Sincerely yours,

Daniel L. Cooper

Daniel L. Cooper
Under Secretary for Benefits

This response was supposed to satisfy my concerns concerning what the VA could or could not do in compiling data. However, twenty days later the secretary's office released a VA fact sheet dated December 2004 in which they boast of their accomplishment in fiscal year 2003. This VA fact sheet demonstrates the VA has the ability to track all incoming claims and how many claims each Regional Office approves. The full fact sheet and a discussion of its implications can be found in chapter 4.

The Appeal Process

There is a definite set of rules that must be observed when a veteran appeals a VA decision denying benefits. The first step is to file a Notice of Disagreement with the Regional Office of original jurisdiction within one year of the date the veteran received the denial letter.

If the issue is not resolved to the veteran's satisfaction by the RO, the case is forwarded to the Board of Veteran's Appeals in Washington. If the BVA ruling has not resolved the issue, the veteran can have his or her case heard before the U.S. Court of Appeals for Veterans Claims. An unsatisfactory decision by this court can be heard before the Federal Circuit Court of Appeals. The last stop in the appeal process is the Supreme Court.

"They Did It Before and They Will Do It Again"

One veteran pursued his claims to the fullest extent and would not give up until the case was argued before the Supreme Court. In its ruling on the case, the Court sided with veteran Fred Gardner, agreeing that he should be paid compensation for the disabilities incurred while a patient of the VA.

Associate Justice Souter, writing for a unanimous Court held

that Paragraph 3.358(c)(3) (38 *CFR*) is not consistent with the plain language of the Title 38 U.S. Code §1151, which does not contain a word about fault or accident. The statutory text and reasonable inferences from it give a clear answer against the Government's arguments that a fault requirement is implicit in the terms "injury" and "as a result of." This clear textually grounded conclusion is also fatal to the Government's remaining principal arguments: that Congress ratified the VA's practice of requiring a showing of fault when it reenacted the predecessor of §1151 in 1934, or, alternatively, that the post-1934 legislative silence serves as an implicit endorsement of the fault based policy; and that the policy deserves judicial deference due to its undisturbed endurance. Pp. 2-8. 5 F. 3d 1456, affirmed.

This practice is no different than the VA adding to its operational manual (M21-1) that to qualify for Direct Service-Connection the veteran must be awarded a Bronze Star or Air Medal with a "V" device. Without aggressive oversight, the VA will continue to implement policies unfair to veterans in the name of reducing budget requirements.

Allen v. Principi: Alcohol Abuse Secondary to PTSD

Veteran William Allen, unsatisfied with the CAVC's decision on his case, took his case to the U.S. Court of Appeals for the Federal Circuit in Washington, and on February 2, 2001, the court decided one of the landmark cases upholding veterans' rights. The finding by the U.S. Circuit Court of Appeals blocked one of the many tactics used by the VA to deny PTSD claims.

FACTS
William Allen served on active duty in the U.S. Marine Corps from September 1965 to September 1969. Mr. Allen alleged that he suffered from PTSD resulting from his service. He also alleged that he suffered from an alcohol abuse disability that manifested itself as a symptom of his PTSD. In 1999, he requested increased monetary compensation for both his PTSD and for his alcohol abuse disability. Mr. Allen challenged the VA's position that the existence of his alcohol abuse disability should be considered in determining his disability rating for PTSD.

HISTORY
In 1993, the Boston Regional Office granted Mr. Allen a 30% disability rating for service-connected PTSD effective from June 1992. In October 1994, Mr. Allen filed a claim for an increased rating. The RO issued a rating decision in June 1995 refusing an increase but confirming the 30% disability rating.

In 1995–96, Dr. Victoria Russell conducted a VA Compensation and Pension examination to determine the severity of Mr. Allen's PTSD and to ascertain whether there was a relationship between Allen's PTSD and his alcohol abuse. Dr. Russell wrote that "the reason for [Allen's] alcohol admissions had to do with his rapidly accelerating symptoms of PTSD." The doctor diagnosed Mr. Allen with severe PTSD in addition to her diagnosis of chronic alcohol abuse and dependence, in remission, secondary to PTSD. In November 1996, the RO issued a rating confirming the 30% disability evaluation for PTSD and again declining an increased rating.

On June 6, 1997, however, following a psychiatric hospitalization, the RO increased Mr. Allen's disability rating to 50%, effective from October 13, 1994. Although the RO considered Mr. Allen's prior hospitalizations in determining his rating, the RO did not consider the August 1996 C&P Exam by Dr. Russell in evaluating whether Mr. Allen was entitled to an increased rating above 50%.

Mr. Allen appealed the denial of a rating higher than 50% to the BVA. On November 26, 1997, the board upheld the RO and denied a higher rating. The board said that "alcohol abuse may not be service-connected, on either a direct or secondary basis, and impairment from non-service-connected substance abuse may not be considered when evaluating the severity of the service-connected PTSD." In order to receive a 70% rating—the next available step above 50%—the board required Mr. Allen to demonstrate both occupational impairment and social impairment.

In considering all of the evidence, the board decided that "the record demonstrates that the veteran's employability has been seriously undermined by his history of alcohol abuse and dependence," but determined that Mr. Allen's PTSD was "not the only factor influencing his industrial [occupational] impairment." The board also found that Mr. Allen failed to produce sufficient evidence to demonstrate social impairment.

On March 25, 1998, Mr. Allen filed a timely appeal to the CAVC. On July 12, 1999, the U.S. Court of Appeals for Veterans Claims vacated the BVA's decision and remanded the case for a further evidentiary hearing. Both Mr. Allen and the secretary of veterans affairs agreed that a remand was required in light of the CAVC's opinion in *Barela v. West*, which had been issued subsequent to the board's November 26, 1997, decision.[1] In *Barela* it was held that U.S. Code §1110 precludes a veteran from receiving compensation for disabilities resulting from alcohol or drug abuse. In its *Barela* ruling, however, the court added that §1110 does not bar an award of service connection for alcohol or drug abuse. An award of service connection would entitle a veteran to benefits such as educational assistance for dependents or housing loan benefits for the veteran. It would not entitle the veteran to any increase in disability compensation.

Initially Mr. Allen appealed to CAVC to vacate the November 26, 1997, BVA decision that denied increased disability compensation. In its one-judge order, the CAVC instructed the board that its interpretation in *Barela v. West* was a *binding precedent* and barred recovery to the extent that Mr. Allen sought increased compensation for his alcohol abuse disability, either as a secondary service-connected disability or as evidence of the increased severity of his service-connected post-traumatic stress disorder.

JUDICIAL APPRAISAL

U.S. Court of Appeals for the Federal Circuit held they have jurisdiction over this remand order because the CAVC interpretation of the statute will affect the remand proceeding, and our future review may be evaded. "We further hold that §1110, when read in light of its legislative history, *does not preclude a veteran from receiving compensation for alcohol or drug-related disabilities arising secondarily from a service-connected disability, or from using alcohol or drug-related disabilities as evidence of the increased severity of a service-connected disability.* Therefore, we reject the CAVC statutory interpretation of §1110 and to that extent reverse the court's order, and remand for proceedings in accordance with the interpretation of §1110 as set forth herein. The part of the order remanding to the Board for proper application of the rating criteria is affirmed." (Italics added.)

In Allen's case, the CAVC remanded in order for the board to apply the court's interpretation of §1110 as set forth in *Barela.* Allen had argued that *Barela* was "wrongly decided to the extent that it held that the law prohibits the payment by VA of compensation for alcohol abuse either on a secondary-service-connection basis or as evidence of an increase in the severity of a service-connected disability." The Court of Appeals for Veterans Claims, however, rejected Mr. Allen's interpretation of §1110 and stated that *Barela* was "binding precedent" to the extent that Mr. Allen "seeks compensation based either on alcohol abuse secondary to service-connected PTSD or an increase in his rating for service-connected PTSD based on manifestations of PTSD symptomatology, i.e., alcohol or drug abuse."

COURT'S RULING

We therefore conclude, based on the language of the statute and the pertinent legislative history, that 38 U.S.C. §1110 does not preclude compensation for an alcohol or drug abuse disability secondary to a service-connected disability or use of an alcohol or drug abuse disability as evidence of the increased severity of a service-connected disability. We would stress that the holding of the case is quite limited. Veterans can only recover if they can adequately establish that their alcohol or drug abuse disability is secondary to or is caused by their primary service-connected disorder. We foresee that such compensation would only result where there is clear medical evidence establishing that the alcohol or drug abuse disability is indeed caused by a veteran's primary service-connected disability, and where the alcohol or drug abuse disability is not due to willful wrongdoing.

On remand, the Board will have to determine whether Allen's alcohol abuse disability is secondary to his PTSD, or whether it demonstrates the increased severity of his PTSD disability. If it finds sufficient evidence demonstrating a causal connection, Allen could be entitled to an increase in his schedular rating. But if the Division Review Officer finds that Allen's alcohol abuse is willful and did not result from his PTSD, Allen could not receive additional compensation for a willful alcohol abuse disability. Barela and any other decisions of the Veterans Court are hereby overruled, to the extent they are contrary to this opinion.

For the foregoing reasons, the decision of the Veterans Court is affirmed-in-part and reversed-in-part. The case is remanded to the Veterans Court for further proceedings consistent with this opinion.

WHAT WE LEARNED
1. A veteran does not have to exhibit both occupational and social impairment before he or she can qualify for PTSD benefits under Diagnostic Code 9411. If you have one or the other diagnosed by a physician, you meet the basic standard. PTSD claims suffer a high casualty rate when it comes time to rate a claim because adjudicators have historically required degrees of proof that are not required by law.
2. Section 1110, 38 U. S. Code does not bar compensation payment for a claim involving alcohol or drug abuse if, in fact, this abuse is a secondary condition brought about by a service-related injury or disease. It also can be used as evidence that the service-connected condition has increased in its severity.

U.S. Court of Appeals for Veterans Claims

The rest of this chapter consists of cases heard by the U.S. Court of Appeals for Veterans Claims. In these cases, the court dealt with questions of substance abuse, noncombat-related PTSD experienced in a combat environment, sexual assault, noncombat MOS in a combat zone, and injury caused by a lighting strike. All of these cases, representing a cross-section of obstacles a veteran faces when he or she files an appeal, touch on a PTSD claimant's needs.

Flayter v. Principi: Substance Abuse

FACTS
In the case of *Flayter v. Principi*, the VA denied benefits based on the finding in *Barela v. West*.[2] When the U.S. Court of Appeals for the Federal Circuit overruled *Barela v. West*, the U.S. Court of Appeals for Veterans Claims gained the authority to reverse the BVA in *Flayter v. Principi*.

Flayter v. Principi is a memorandum decision (single-judge ruling), which means it cannot be cited as an authority in an appeal to the court.[3] It is, however, extremely valuable for a veteran who is filing a claim based on alcohol or substance abuse as secondary to PTSD. The good news is *William F. Allen v. Anthony J. Principi*,[4] when appealed to the U.S. Court of Appeals for the Federal Circuit, overturned *Barela v. West*. In *Allen v. Principi* the VA rubber-stamped the denial letters where alcohol or substance abuse was secondary to PTSD. A decision by the U.S. Court of Appeals for the Federal Circuit can be cited in a case on appeal before the U.S. Court of Appeals for Veterans Claims.

HISTORY
In 1996 Mr. Patrick Flayter filed a claim for increased disability compensation in excess of 30% for PTSD and service connection for alcohol and drug abuse secondary to PTSD. The RO denied his claim in May 1997 for increased compensation for PTSD. Flayter was granted service connection for drug and alcohol abuse secondary to PTSD. However, in this case, claims examiners denied paying compensation for drug and alcohol abuse. They cited statutes that they say prohibit payment for any condition caused by willful misconduct on the part of the veteran. They maintained *Barela v. West* prevailed in Mr. Flayter's case, thus denying compensation payment for alcohol and drug abuse secondary to PTSD.

JUDICIAL REVIEW
The veteran filed a timely appeal of the denial of increased compensation with CAVC, and a decision was rendered approximately two and a half years later on April 7, 2001. CAVC reversed the BVA based on the findings announced by the Federal Court of Appeals for the Federal District in their decision of *Allen v. Principi*, Docket Number 98 555, decided on April 11, 2002.[5]

The crux of this case was that a veteran can receive compensation for an alcohol or drug abuse disability where it is established that such a disability is secondary to or is caused by his or her primary disability or disorder. This decision does not limit the scope of secondary alcohol or drug abuse to only PTSD.

COURT'S RULING
In view of the finding in *Allen v. Principi*, the court vacated the BVA decision and remanded it back to be readjudicated consistent with this order.

WHAT WE LEARNED
1. When the Court of Appeals for Veterans Claims renders a single-judge decision, you cannot use it as an instrument to force the VA to change its finding in your case. Only issues addressed by a three-judge panel can be quoted as law, thus forcing the VA to comply with its decision. However, a single-judge finding (referred to as a memorandum decision) can be valuable to you if you use it as a tool to frame your claim before the VA.
2. Once again the Department of Veterans Affairs's administrative function is forced to change its policy to conform to the law. It is almost certain if Flayter's claim was decided a year earlier by the CAVC, the decision would not have been vacated and the veteran would not have had a second bite out of the apple. It never pays to leave a denied claim unchallenged. When the VA denies your claim, file a Notice of Disagreement within a year of the date you were notified.

3. The decision by the U.S. Court of Appeals for the Federal Circuit stopped the VA from denying compensation benefits when alcohol or substance abuse is secondary to PTSD. Prior to this decision claims examiners would grant service connection for this secondary condition, but would withhold compensation stating it was the result of willful misconduct.

Yancey v. Principi: Noncombat PTSD in a Combat Zone

FACTS
Alberta Yancy's claim for service-connected PTSD benefits was denied by the Board of Veterans Appeals in October 2002. Her case was reviewed before a single judge, making it off limits as a precedent-mandating authority. Even so, this case can show you what to do and what not to do.[6]

HISTORY
Ms. Yancy, the appellant, served on active duty in the U.S. Army from December 1990 to May 1991 during Operations Desert Shield and Desert Storm. The record shows she was stationed in Saudi Arabia from January to May 1991. She was a practical nurse attached to the 114th Evacuation Hospital Unit. In a supplemental medical report dated May 1991, Ms. Yancy was asked whether she experienced insomnia, interrupted sleep, or dreams about war experiences. She was quoted as saying, "I have nightmares of gerbils holding me down" and a "fear of getting hit by a scud." In another record, a sick call record dated April 1991, she told the doctor "she was having nightmares when she first arrived in country." Her record notes "reoccurring thoughts about her experiences in Saudi Arabia."

In February 1994 the VA ordered a C&P examination following her application for compensation benefits. The C&P examiner reported:

> She had flashbacks of "many scuds" coming close. The claimant stated that there were days when there were four scud attacks per day. . . . She is reminded and relives some intrusive memories of the scud attacks when she sees trucks or dollies.

The examiner diagnosed the appellant with PTSD, delayed. During that same month, the VA scheduled her for a C&P social survey, part of the C&P examination for PTSD that determines the veteran's ability to work in the public domain. The examiner reported, while on active duty, the appellant had "begun becoming more terrified as scud missiles struck close to 114th Evacuation Hospital Unit compound. It was here that she began periods of restlessness and poor sleep."

In February 1994 a statement in support of claim (VA Form 21-4138) was filed with the VA Regional Office. The record shows she stated that she "had been very fearful of the scud missiles." In June 1994 the RO issued a decision in which it denied the appellant's PTSD claim. The RO decided her "unverified general statements about being afraid of the scud missile attacks are not acceptable evidence of an incident or incidents during active service which would cause PTSD."

On March 2, 1995, the veteran filed a notice to reopen her claim based on new and material evidence. In that statement, she commented, "Being a nurse by profession I somewhat understand why the claim was denied. But, by the same token working as a fulltime professional nurse, I don't understand why a person my age should be under constant medical care, taking daily medication." She requested that the RO obtain her most recent medical records for a "new evaluation." Ms. Yancy also reported that many symptoms related to her several disabilities (for which she was claiming service connection), including PTSD, had been exacerbated.

The court noted that the RO and the BVA treated this March 1995 VA Form 21-4138 as an attempt to reopen a previously disallowed claim. Subsequently, the RO requested copies of the appellant's private medical records. This was followed in April 1995 by an order for another C&P general evaluation and a PTSD examination.

The April 1995 PTSD examination report acknowledged that the veteran was preoccupied with memories of scud missile attacks and offered a diagnosis of borderline PTSD. The October 1995 PTSD examination report diagnosed the appellant with PTSD, "borderline, by history only," and chronic major depression. The RO, in August 1995, requested the appellant's service records from the commander of the U.S. Army Reserve Unit. The request for background information included the veteran's unit and dates of assignment and participation in combat operations during Desert Storm. The court notes it appears that the RO did not receive this information. In November 1995, the RO requested a DA Form 20, a Department of the Army personnel record of the soldier's history, from the U.S. Army Reserve Personnel Center. It was further noted by the court that the Records on Appeal did not contain a copy of any such form or file.

The VA claims examiners rated her claim for PTSD in February 1996, reaffirming the denial of her PTSD claim. She appealed that decision in March 1996 by filing a Notice of Disagreement. In March 1996 the VA responded with a Statement of the Case.

The veteran was given a hearing before the local RO's hearing officer in July 1996 where she testified that there had been three to four scud missile attacks every night during the three weeks that she had been stationed in Dhahran, Saudi Arabia. Ms. Yancy also testified that she treated wounded allied personnel and enemy prisoners of war. She further testified that, after service, certain noises and odors had triggered flashbacks and the nightmares that she had begun to experience in Saudi Arabia had worsened. Her representative indicated that the appellant anticipated obtaining personally her DA Form 20 from her Army Reserve Unit in St. Louis, Missouri. However, the ROA does not reflect that the appellant submitted any such request.

As noted in a December 1996 VA Treatment Summary, the veteran reported stressful events occurred while she was serving on active duty. These events included: (1) hearing "constant" warning sirens used to alert personnel of missile attacks, (2) "constantly" getting in and out of protective chemical warfare gear and being afraid of chemical exposure while she slept, (3) witnessing a child die from a heart condition, (4) talking with an Enemy Prisoner of War (EPW) whose arm had been amputated, (5) hearing gunfire in the compound, (6) learning of her mother's heart attack and of her grandmother's death, and (7) merging with another unit prior to activation.

In September 1997 the RO received from a veteran who had served with the appellant a statement that during service the appellant had been subjected to "additional pressures due to emergencies at home"; the appellant had made "three trips back to the United States" prompted by family emergencies, including one leave of approximately three weeks.

In a September 1998 decision, the BVA determined that the record confirmed the appellant had a diagnosis of PTSD, but that she had not engaged in combat with the enemy. Based on the latter determination, the board stated VA regulations required the appellant's alleged stressors be corroborated by credible supporting evidence. The board concluded that the record lacked credible supporting evidence and thus it remanded the matter and ordered that the RO: (1) "attempt to obtain copies of the action reports or unit histories" for the appellant's unit and (2) "make a determination as to whether any of the [appellant's] claimed stressors are verified by these unit histories."

Subsequently the RO requested from the U.S. Armed Services Center for Research of Unit Records (USASCRUR) copies of the veteran's unit historical records from January to May 1991. The RO claims examiner explained it was "trying to determine if the veteran's unit was attacked by scud missiles on several occasions."

In June 1999 USASCRUR responded by providing the RO with a unit history submitted by the 114th that "documents the locations, missions, operations and significant activities of the unit during the veteran's tour of duty." The unit history report, dated March 15, 1991, reflects that the 114th spent its first three weeks of deployment in "transient quarters in Dhahran, Saudi Arabia, before establishing its evacuation hospital near King Khalid Military City, Saudi Arabia." The report also reflects that: (1) a public address system was "necessary for enemy threat alerts," (2) Purple Hearts were awarded to three members of the unit, (3) the unit treated large numbers of wounded EPWs, and (4) the "unit was in danger in Dhahran without proper protection during scud attacks."

Following receipt of this report, the RO claims examiners issued a Supplemental SOC in which they continued the denial of her PTSD claim. The RO justified denying her claim:

> The unit history noted the existence of enemy threat and also noted that the unit was in danger in Dhahran. However, it failed to note any actual scud attack on the

114th Evacuation Hospital location. There is no information on the frequency of these attacks or the severity that may have followed the attacks.

The SSOC made no mentioning or offered any documentation of the wounded. They concluded the evidence reviewed still did not verify the stressful experiences that the veteran claimed.

In October 2000 the veteran rejected the decision of the BVA and on February 10, 2001, filed a timely Notice of Appeal to the U.S. Court of Appeals for Veterans Claims. Her brief filed with the court challenged the BVA decision denying benefits.

JUDICIAL REVIEW

The board members concluded that the 114th's unit history report did not provide evidence sufficient to corroborate her reported stressor of experiencing multiple scud missile attacks. The BVA made the point that the report did "not state the veteran's unit actually came under attack by scuds, nor did it state the frequency or duration of these attacks." The board further stated, although some of the appellant's other alleged stressors were verifiable, all of her diagnoses of PTSD were based on the alleged in-service stressor related to scud missile attacks. Thus, the board concluded none of her PTSD diagnoses were linked to a specific in-service stressor, verified by credible supporting evidence; therefore they denied her claim for service connection for PTSD.

COURT'S RULING

Chief Judge Kramer stated he was not prepared to rule on the question of the quantum of evidence that the unit history report provides as to whether the 114th actually came under attack or attacks from scud missiles. The court's discretion allows for a remand on such matter.

The court ordered on remand the VA should attempt to secure documents that provide detail regarding the appellant's duty stations, dates of assignments, and dates of the appellant's physical presence at the location of the 114th. Moreover, the court further noted that the unit history report reflects that the "unit was in danger in Dhahran without proper protection during scud attacks," but that it does not provide any detail about any actual attack that occurred between January and March 15, 1991. The court noted that, as of March 15, 1991, according the unit history report, the 114th was no longer in Dhahran, Saudi Arabia, the location where the appellant maintains that she had experienced her scud-missile stressor. On remand, the VA should attempt to obtain specific information as to whether and when any such attack actually occurred while the veteran was physically present at the 114th's location. In the event that further army documents are unavailable, the VA should survey unit members as to these inquiries. Further, the board is directed on remand to address the effect of the words "during scud attacks" and the significance of the three Purple Hearts awarded to members of the 114th.

Finally, on remand the appellant is free to submit additional evidence and argument, including those arguments raised in her briefs to this court. The board shall proceed expeditiously, in accordance with 38 U.S.C. 7112.

WHAT WE LEARNED

Alberta Yancey's case is an excellent example of a delaying tact by the Department of Veterans Affairs. Ms. Yancy doggedly held on for more than twelve years and deserves many kudos for not letting the process force her to cave in. She has persisted and used the system, expecting the VA to consider all the information necessary to process her claim.

Unfortunately, she is now twelve years down the road and no closer to having her award granted. Even though the law mandates that adjudicators assist in developing the claim, provided the claim is well grounded, they have not fulfilled their duty to assist.

In this case the court raised issues it expects the VA to act upon. Unless the evidence is indisputable, a VA adjudicator will deny a veteran's claim. In other words, if you cannot force the VA to grant benefits by introducing solid evidence, you'll be unsuccessful during the first round. If a claim is based on either the claimant's combat with the enemy or rape, the chances are it will be approved. Title 38 *USC*, chapter 51, section 5103A, leaves options open as far as the VA's duty to assist. An adjudicator must make only a *reasonable effort* to assist a claimant, and he or she is not required to assist if, in his or her opinion, the claim cannot be proved.

You can learn from *Yancey v. Principi* and take steps that will help you file a winning claim:

1. Have all statements from former members sworn and notarized. These documents now become evidence that cannot be dismissed as unsubstantiated statements.
2. If the unit history report does not support your statement, then try to obtain a report from the next level of command, which summarizes events occurring in all its suborganizations.
3. Do not hesitate to involve your congressional representative or senator in expediting your request for records.
4. Remember you can be your own advocate. I mean no disrespect to all the service officers' nationwide, but they have not been trained to be aggressive advocates. The VA basically uses these service officers as clerks, but few service officers know what the law requires when documenting hundreds of details into binding evidence.

Doran v. Brown: Noncombat Disability— A Lighting Bolt from Zeus

FACTS

I have selected the *Doran v. Brown* case for further discussion because it demonstrates the kind of review a PTSD claim undergoes when the circumstances fail to fit a narrow definition of PTSD.[7] It appears that the only PTSD claims that have a chance of being granted have a combat incident or rape as the stressor. Many cases have come before the court that reflect how the intent of Congress is ultimately manipulated by simply changing the wording in VA manuals.

The court gave veterans claiming PTSD caused by noncombat-related stressors a leg up when it decided Robert Doran's case. The court closed the door on one of the VA's most frequently used reasons for denying claims: "the absence of support in service records."

HISTORY

In 1976 Robert E. Doran reopened his claim for psychoneurosis to include post-traumatic stress disorder, based on new and material evidence. However, it wasn't until August 1992 that his case made its way through the system to the court for the first time. When he reopened his claim and the court heard his case in 1993, he submitted medical evidence from the doctor who treated him for his neurosis and PTSD. He was also able to obtain lay statements from individuals who were knowledgeable of the circumstance of his stressors.

Mr. Doran claimed that during his active service (1950–1952) he was struck by lighting, causing unconsciousness and requiring resuscitation. The second stressor cited by Mr. Doran was an encounter with a snake on an infiltration course. The court considered the evidence submitted in support of his claim noncumulative, not relevant to or probative to the issue at hand. On August 7, 1992, the court issued a single-judge memorandum decision vacating the Board of Veterans' Appeals' November 28, 1990, denial of service connection and remanded it back to the VA for readjudication.

JUDICIAL APPRAISAL

The court held that the "board focused only on evidence that tended to support the denial of service connection, ignored evidence in favor of the appellant's claim, and failed to provide reasons or basis for its findings and conclusions." The order further stipulated, on remand, the board would adjudicate Mr. Doran's claim for service connection for PTSD, a claim that was raised but not addressed by the VA.

On March 5, 1993, the Board of Veterans' Appeals issued a decision in which they determined (1) the evidence received by the VA since the BVA denied entitlement for service connection for a psychoneurosis in September 1976 was both new and material and the claim for psychoneurosis to include PTSD would be reopened; (2) the veteran's psychoneurosis preexisted active service and the sound condition at enlistment had been rebutted; (3) the psychoneurosis was not aggravated during service; and (4) service connection for PTSD was not warranted. Mr. Doran filed a timely appeal to the court.

One year later, on March 8, 1994, a three-judge panel heard Mr. Doran's appeal to the court. That portion of the court's discussion and decision concerning the aggravation of a preexisting psychoneurotic condition will not be addressed as it is not pertinent to establishing service connection for PTSD.

The court found that the BVA's treatment of Mr. Doran's claim for PTSD highlighted the potential inconsistency between the statute, the regulations, and the specific provisions of VA Adjudication Manual "M21-1." The court clarified the section of the manual that required "service records must support the assertion that the veteran was subjected to a stressor of sufficient gravity to evoke symptoms (PTSD) in almost anyone." The court held that under the governing statutory and regulatory provisions regarding claims for service connection for PTSD, "if the claimed stressor is not combat-related, appellant's lay testimony regarding in service stressors is insufficient to establish the occurrence of the stressor and must be corroborated by credible supporting evidence. . . . *There is nothing in the stature or the regulations which provides that corroboration must and can only be found in service records.*" (Italics added.) Those service records that are available must not contradict the appellant's lay testimony concerning his noncombat stressor. *VA manuals cannot give out instructions, which are contrary to the statute.*

COURT'S RULING
For the second time the court vacated the VA's decision to deny benefits. Mr. Doran's case was remanded with instruction to readjudicate his claim for PTSD making certain that a critical examination is conducted of all the evidence when justifying the decision. Because Robert Doran does not appear in public records, it is not known if the VA has readjudicated his claim for PTSD and granted the benefits or whether the local rating board has continued to deny his claim, thus forcing him to continue with the appeal process.

WHAT WE LEARNED
This case opened the door exposing many of the tactics that are used by various rating officers. If the circumstances of your appeal can be supported by the finding in this case, it can be cited because it is a three-judge decision. Here are several key points to keep in mind when preparing your claim or if you are appealing any denial of benefits:

1. The VA cannot publish a change to its manuals that is contrary to the statutes. Be alert for this. This is why you should do your research before you submit a claim.
2. There is nothing in the law or regulations that requires corroboration of a traumatic event to come from service records.
3. The court recognized a potential inconsistency between the statutes, regulations and the specific provisions in VA Manual M-21-1.

Patton v. West: Sexual Assault

FACTS

The case of *Dorrance H. Patton v. Togo D. West* demonstrates many of the problems encountered by an individual who was traumatized by an noncombat-related event, which then took thirty-three years to surface as PTSD.[7] You will note as you read Judge Steinberg's account of the events that Mr. Patton initially was diagnosed with anxiety and depressive neurosis; emotional instability reaction, chronic, moderate, manifested by diffused anxiety; and poor performance under stress. These conditions were the reason he was found unfit for duty and given an honorable administrative discharge.

HISTORY

The veteran served in the U.S. Army from March to August 1956 and from October 1959 until February 1960. His service medical records (SMRs) indicated normal psychiatric clinical evaluations at the time of his first entry into service, first discharge, and second entrance physical.

On the evening of December 9, 1959, the veteran was admitted to the emergency room of an army hospital, where he was treated for an acute anxiety reaction. A detailed description of his treatment contained notations that he was afraid someone would "jump him" and that "inferentially, his profound feelings of shame, as well as other indirect derivatives suggest to me that there may be underlying homosexual panic." The SMRs also indicated that he complained of headaches, anorexia, and sleeplessness, and that he attributed "most of his problems" to an incident when he had been hit in the head with a glass bottle while on leave a few weeks before. According to those records, other soldiers in the barracks reported that the veteran had "some sort of attack" the night he was first admitted to the army hospital. Although SMRs dated December 10, 1959, report his anxiety appeared to have worsened since he had arrived at Fort Bragg, the ROA contains no notations of anxiety prior to December 9, 1959.

The veteran's service personnel records contain no indication of any in-service assault incident. On January 21, 1960, "despite a limited work assignment," the veteran "presented himself in a tearful disheveled state" at the army hospital. He was diagnosed as having "emotional instability reaction, chronic, moderate; manifested by diffuse anxiety, poor performance under stress, and administrative separation from the service [was] recommended." During 1978 and 1979 the veteran was hospitalized several times in a VA medical facility, was treated for anxiety and depressive neurosis, and received medication from VA and psychotherapy from a private clinic. In August 1978 he reported a history of alcoholism and in March 1979 he "admitted to heavy use of alcohol as a means of coping with his anxiety" and was diagnosed by a VA psychiatrist as having a paranoid personality.

In May 1979 a VA physician diagnosed the veteran as having a "habitual excessive drinking" disorder and stated: "On previous admission patient had been called paranoid type personality though at this time I feel that this is probably this patient's basic underlying personality type which was brought out by his decompensation due to many years of alcohol abuse." The veteran submitted letters from two acquaintances; each provided general information about his nervous condition and requested any assistance the VA could provide for the veteran. One mentioned the veteran's drinking problem.

The veteran also submitted an August 1979 letter from his wife detailing his changed behavior since service, including his "not getting along with people, . . . his hiding behind his drinking, . . . his anger and depression, and his being ashamed of the way he was. . . . She specifically reported that around the end of 1961, the veteran's mother had written to her saying . . . she was afraid he might kill himself and that . . . something had happened to him in the service."

The veteran submitted a July 1979 letter from a private physician stating that the veteran was "extremely agitated, depressed, loses control of his temper, and was potentially dangerous to both himself and others," and had been so for the prior twelve months. The physician also stated that the veteran had not responded to medication and other treatments and he might "lose control and kill someone."

In September 1979, after the VA Regional Office denied service connection for a nervous condition and sent the veteran a Statement of the Case, the veteran filed a VA Form 1-9, Substantive Appeal to the BVA. At an October 1979 hearing at the RO regarding the nervous-condition claim, the veteran testified under oath that he had been hospitalized after an altercation with a noncommissioned officer; that he did not "know what in the hell happened: it just all went black"; that he had then received a medical discharge of which he was ashamed; that since he left the service he had "done a lot of heavy drinking to cover this up"; that his anxiety had become worse since he stopped drinking a few years ago; and that, until recently, he had not sought psychiatric assistance because he did not want anyone to know about his problem. He subsequently submitted both VA and private medical records from 1976 through 1981, including a January 1981 private psychiatric evaluation that noted that the veteran had "a paranoid personality with decompensation into a psychotic state manifested by homicidal ideation, agitation and depression." No BVA decision apparently was issued in connection with the 1979 RO denial. The ROA does not reflect further contact with the VA by the veteran until 1993.

When the error was found in 1993, a C&P examination was scheduled. During the November 1993 VA medical examination, the veteran stated, for the first time to any medical professional, that while he was at Fort Bragg, he had been raped by three men and that he did not report it because of "fear and shame." He disclosed that after a second hospitalization (apparently in January 1960) he had told a sergeant about the rape and that the sergeant had instructed him not to tell anyone. At that time he was diagnosed, for the first time, with "*PTSD, non-combat, chronic.*"(Italics added.)

In December 1993 the veteran sought to have his nervous-condition claim "reopened to include PTSD." In January 1994, a VA medical examiner diagnosed PTSD, clearly relating the PTSD to the alleged in-service rape trauma. In December 1994 the RO denied service connection for PTSD, finding that the veteran had not provided the required corroborating evidence for an in-service, noncombat stressor.

The veteran appealed to the board in a timely manner. In April 1995, he testified under oath before the RO that he had been sexually assaulted, but had been told (presumably by a sergeant) that he would receive a dishonorable discharge and would be sent to prison if he reported it. In the 1997 BVA decision on appeal, the board denied the PTSD claim because it was "based on non-combat-related unverified stressors," and because corroboration of an in-service stressor was an essential element of the veteran's PTSD claim.

MOTION TO STRIKE

The first issue the court had to address was a motion to strike by the Department of Veterans Affairs. The veteran contended that, in the absence of evidence of a combat-related stressor, he must "furnish the specific details of the in-service incident." He stated that he has "attempted to submit an affidavit which is confirmed by a third party immediately after this witness left the service."

The secretary responded with a motion to strike references to the affidavit. The court noted that "there is no such exhibit attached to the appellant's brief." In addition, "the court is precluded by statute from including in the Records Contained on Appeal (RCA) any material that was not contained in the record of proceedings before the Secretary and the Board." The court made it known it would not consider the appellant's purported attempt to submit an affidavit as an exhibit to his brief. The order went on to say "the veteran was free to submit additional evidence, including the asserted statement referred to above, to the BVA in connection with the remand that the court ordered in its opinion."

This is an important point to remember if your claim goes to the CAVC. Once the BVA has reviewed your appeal, no new evidence can be added to the file by either side. However, if your claim is remanded back to the controlling Regional Office, you can add new evidence for them to consider. If the BVA affirms the local RO decision to deny benefits, the case must go as is to the court with no new evidence attached.

COURT'S RULING

Judge Steinberg, writing for the majority, presented a fast moving account of the events that reshaped Mr. Patton's life. Judge Holdaway did not agree with the majority decision, and thus filed a dissenting opinion.

The court's finding for this case laid out a great set of basic rules the veteran and VA must observe. The court's decision in this case has provided us with eight rules to build a solid claim for service-connected PTSD:

1. The third rule outlines exactly what the court will look for should you challenge the VA's denial of benefits. The veteran must show the following key points:
   - a current, clear, medical diagnosis of PTSD;
   - credible supporting evidence that the claimed in-service stressor actually occurred;
   - medical evidence of a causal connection between current symptomatology and the specific, claimed, in-service stressor. The evidence required to support the occurrence of an in-service stressor varies "depending on whether or not the veteran was engaged in combat with the enemy."
2. The board is required to include in its decision a written statement of the reasons or bases for its findings and conclusions on all material issues of fact and law presented on the record.
3. The VA's statement must adequately enable an appellant to understand the precise basis for the board's decision, as well as facilitate review in the CAVC. To comply with this requirement, the board must analyze the credibility and probative value of the evidence, account for the evidence that it finds to be persuasive or unpersuasive, and provide the reasons for its rejection of any material evidence favorable to the veteran.

   This requirement is one of the most neglected instructions as the VA seldom follows it. Instead claims examiners dismiss a claim by stating that a preponderance of evidence is against the claimant's claim. However, the court ruled the VA must cite "chapter and verse" what evidence is superior to the evidence the claimant submitted. They must also provide an explanation why the evidence favorable to you was not sufficient to grant you benefits.

4.　The evidence required to support the occurrence of an in-service stressor varies "depending on whether or not the veteran was 'engaged in combat with the enemy.'" According to *Zarycki v. Brown,* when the VA determines that the veteran did not engage in combat with the enemy, "the veteran's lay testimony, by itself, will not be enough to establish the occurrence of the alleged stressor."[8] The necessary additional evidence may be obtained from sources other than the veteran's SMRs.

5.　When the law or regulation changes after a claim has been filed or reopened, but not before the administrative or judicial appeal process has been concluded, the version most favorable to the appellant will apply unless Congress legislates otherwise.

6.　The service record may be devoid of evidence because many victims of personal assault, especially sexual assault and domestic violence, do not file official reports either with military or civilian authorities. Therefore, development of alternative sources for information is critical. Alternative sources that may provide credible evidence of the in-service stressor include:

(a) medical records from private (civilian) physicians or caregivers who may have treated the veteran either immediately following the incident or sometime later

(b) civilian police reports

(c) reports from crisis intervention centers such as rape crisis centers or centers for domestic abuse.

7.　Rating board personnel must carefully evaluate all the available evidence. If the military record contains no documentation that a personal assault occurred, alternative evidence might still establish an in-service stressful incident. Behavior changes that occurred at the time of the incident may indicate the occurrence of an in-service stressor. Examples of behavior changes that might indicate a stressor include, but are not limited to:

(a) visits to medical or counseling clinic or dispensary without a specific diagnosis or specific ailment

(b) sudden requests that the veteran's military occupational series or duty assignment be changed without other justification

(c) lay statements describing episodes of depression, panic attacks, or anxiety without an identifiable reasons for the episodes

(d) evidence of substance abuse of alcohol or drugs.

8.　Rating boards may rely on the preponderance of evidence to support their conclusions even if the record does not contain direct contemporary evidence. In personal assault claims, secondary evidence may need interpretation by a clinician, especially if it involves behavior changes. Evidence that documents such behavior changes may require interpretation to clarify its relationship to the medical diagnosis by a VA neuropsychiatric physician.

WHAT WE LEARNED

The most important points in this case are the eight rules stressed by CAVC. They are, in brief:

1. If you appeal, the CAVC will look for medical evidence of PTSD, evidence of an in-service stressor, and evidence that supports a link between the two.
2. The VA's decision must include detailed reasons and basis.
3. The VA must make it clear to the claimant what evidence would support the claim.
4. Evidence must support an in-service occurrence.
5. When the law is changed, the veteran's claim should be evaluated with the version most beneficial to him or her.
6. Service records do not always contain supporting evidence.
7. ROs must evaluate all evidence, both for and against, when deciding a claim.
8. ROs may rely on preponderance of evidence when there is no direct contemporary evidence.

Zarycki v. Brown: In Combat—Wrong MOS

FACTS

Cases such as *Alex E. Zarycki v. Jesse Brown* undoubtedly have played over and over again since 1961. Alex Zarycki's military occupational specialty was a noninfantry designation. Because of his MOS, according to the RO rating board, his alleged PTSD was not caused by participating in actual combat. I suppose you could say he was just in the neighborhood. I ask you, who ever heard of a *wireman* and *switch board operator* working in a hot war zone? His case is as follows.[9]

HISTORY

Mr. Zarycki served on active duty in the U.S. Army from September 1967 to June 1970. From February 1968 to February 1969, he was a member of Headquarters Battery, 7th Battalion, 15th Artillery Brigade, stationed in the Republic of Vietnam. From April to September 1969, the appellant was assigned to Fort Hood, Texas. From September 1969 to June 1970, appellant was reassigned to the Vietnam Theater as a member of Headquarters and Headquarters Company, Second Battalion, 22nd Infantry Brigade, 25th Infantry Division.

The appellant's military occupational specialties are listed as field wireman and switch operator. The appellant received the National Defense Service Medal, the Vietnam Service Medal, the Army Commendation Medal, and the Vietnam Campaign Medal. Both his enlistment and separation examinations were negative for any psychiatric disorders.

In April 1983, the appellant filed an application for compensation for PTSD with a VA Regional Office. On the application form, the veteran noted that he had experienced flashbacks about Vietnam and dreams of dead bodies. In support of his application, he submitted a summary of his hospitalization at a VA medical facility from April 15–21, 1983.

According to the summary by a medical staff member at the VA hospital, Mr. Zarycki was admitted to the VA medical facility because of fear of losing control, depression, and poor impulse control resulting from the stress accompanying his impending divorce. It was noted that the appellant had a history of alcohol and drug abuse, financial difficulties, difficulty in finding employment, and domestic violence. Although the veteran had reported experiencing flashbacks and nightmares, none were reported during the period of hospitalization.

Also noted in the hospitalization summary was "the appellant's criminal history, including stealing, breaking and entering, robbery, and shoplifting. The treating physician commented that the veteran was cooperative, somewhat anxious, trying to impress 'him' with the severity of his Vietnam experiences and how dangerous he could be, showing poor impulse control with a lot of underlying hostility. Basically he appeared to be an angry person who felt that the government owed him something and that he was fundamentally different from the rest of the patients."

In July 1983, the appellant filed a second application for compensation for PTSD with the RO; in describing the nature and history of his disability, he reported that he was experiencing flashbacks, nightmares, detachment, anger, and memory impairment. In September 1983, the RO sent a letter to the claimant requesting that he provide detailed information regarding specific incidents in service that he believed were related to his current psychiatric disorder. That same month, the appellant underwent a VA special neuropsychiatric examination.

In relating the appellant's military and medical history, the examining neuropsychiatrist, Dr. S. Loeb, noted in part:

> The veteran was in the Army from September of 1967 to June of 1970. He was in Vietnam for 2 years, in Cambodia, with the 25th Infantry, in 1970 and later with the 2d Battalion, 22nd Infantry, Mechanized. He worked S-5 Intelligence and Reconnaissance.
>
> In 1968 he was in a three-quarter track vehicle and ended up in a rice paddy. He was unconscious for minutes. He doesn't know of having a skull fracture, had a laceration, did not receive a Purple Heart, but did get medals.

He had the Bronze Star for performing above and beyond the call of duty, in a firefight. He has nightmares twice daily, wakes up in cold sweats. His wife, he dreams, is in a "hooch" and there are 2 squads of MVA [sic] coming toward him and he has no ammunition in his weapon. He sees friends that were killed. A friend named Keith got killed. An RPG put a hole in his head.

He has flashbacks every day. One was triggered off by holes that he saw in the aluminum siding, reminding him of wounds and the firefights connected with them. He was placed in a rice paddy. He feels guilty about surviving, feels guilty about killing innocent people, but he isn't sure that he did, because he couldn't actually see who was killed.

Dr. Loeb rendered a diagnosis of "PTSD in a person with substance use, alcohol and mixed drugs and history of emotional instability, with considerable anxiety and depression."

VA RATING OF THE CLAIM
In a rating decision dated October 1988, the RO denied service connection for PTSD. The RO noted: "Post-traumatic stress disorder has been diagnosed on VA examination, but the diagnosis is not supported by any confirmed stressors or Vietnam experiences, by the evidence of record."

In response and to support his claim, the veteran submitted copies of his criminal records. (People who suffer PTSD are likely to engage in criminal behavior.) In December 1988, the RO again denied service connection for PTSD, finding that no new factual evidence had been presented to warrant service connection for post-traumatic stress disorder or any other condition, as "criminal behavior and difficulties with the justice system resulting from criminal behavior do not constitute an adequate stressor for the grant of service connection for PTSD."

On November 8, 1989, the RO received the appellant's Notice of Disagreement with the denial of his claim for service connection for PTSD. In January 1990, the RO provided the veteran with a Statement of the Case and he perfected an appeal to the BVA shortly thereafter. In October 1990, the appellant's service representative presented oral arguments for subsequent presentation to and review by the BVA. In a decision dated December 11, 1990, the BVA remanded the appellant's claim to the RO for further evidentiary development and readjudication. Prior to readjudication, the board specifically directed:

1.   The veteran should be asked to submit a detailed statement regarding the traumatic events that he claims to have experienced in Vietnam, including names of others involved, units, dates, and so on. He should also be asked to submit the citation for his claimed Bronze Star Medal, since that award is not

shown in his service personnel records. If adequate information is received, it should be forwarded to the U.S. Army and Joint Services Environmental Support Group in Washington, DC for verification.

2. The veteran should be given a comprehensive examination by a board of two psychiatrists to determine the nature and extent of any psychiatric disabilities that he may have. The doctors should perform "psychological studies with post-traumatic stress disorder subscales." All complaints and objective findings should be reported in detail. The claims folder should be made available to the examiners for their review prior to the examination. It is essential that the claims folder be reviewed before a final diagnosis is made, with attention to the police record submitted by appellant.

In January 1991 the RO sent a letter requesting the additional information regarding the veteran's in-service stressors and his Bronze Star Medal, as directed by the BVA in its December 1990 decision.

In February 1991 Mr. Zarycki underwent another VA special neuropsychiatric examination; the examination was conducted by one psychiatrist rather than by a board of two psychiatrists as had been directed by the BVA. The examining psychiatrist, Dr. G. A. Batizy, noted that "appellant was not hallucinatory or delusional, but he showed elevated expansive mood with definite liability, also he had over-talkative-ness, destructibility, and flight of ideas. He was also overtly anxious when he was talking about his Vietnam experiences. Intellectually, he was functioning fairly well. His memory was intact to remote and recent events. However, due to his disorganized thinking, both his insight and judgment were definitely distorted."

Dr. Batizy diagnosed the veteran with bipolar disorder, mixed moderate; PTSD; alcohol abuse; and cannabis abuse. Approximately one week later, the appellant underwent a battery of psychological tests. The administering psychologist, Dr. William F. Flynn, reported:

Reality contact has weak spots, with some perceptions blocked, at least initially, some distorted, and some peculiar ideation present. Lying just beneath the surface is a great store of combat/mayhem themes. When stimuli in the environment touch on this, veteran could lose his judgment, impulse control, and even orientation, with resultant violence. He therefore keeps interaction to a minimum.

Reinforcing the trend toward isolation is paranoid component, involving the belief that et al. former co-workers were against him because of his Vietnam history, as well as jealousy on their part. He is also subject to auditory hallucinations in which drill instructors tell him he loves no one, and should kill. He seeks refuge from his conflicts in excessive fantasy, which only strengthens people's perception of him as "weird." Obsessive rumination and a high level of tension make normal functioning difficult if not impossible. He is currently depressed in the mild range, and suicidal ideas are entertained at times, but the act is presently forestalled by concern for his son.

Dr. Flynn concluded that appellant's test record was "consistent with a picture of PTSD superimposed on Bipolar Disorder Not Otherwise Specified."

Thereafter, the veteran submitted a detailed statement recounting his experiences in Vietnam and Cambodia. He reported that approximately two weeks after arriving in Vietnam in 1968, he saw a pile of dead enemy soldiers, which made him unable to eat for four days. He described a "wave" infantry attack at landing zone Crystal. He claimed during his first tour of duty in Vietnam, a fellow serviceman, Private First Class Wake, committed suicide behind the motor pool at LZ Uplift.

The veteran also alleged that his unit was ambushed by sniper fire between LZ Pony and LZ Uplift, and that the bullets came between himself and a friend. He claimed that during his second tour of duty in Vietnam, he worked in communications for S-5 Intelligence. He alleged that he was involved in reconnaissance missions into Cambodia and during one such mission, the vehicle in which he was riding was ambushed resulting in several casualties and injuries. He stated that in June 1970, a fellow soldier, identified only as "Keith," wrote to his son in West Virginia telling him that he would be returning home in thirty days and would take him fishing. Keith then was killed shortly after writing the letter.

The veteran also claimed that an unidentified fellow soldier received stomach wounds from flying shrapnel, while another "had his ear drums blown out." He also described how a medic in his unit was injured in the crotch by flying shrapnel. He reported that a personal friend of his, Sergeant Webb, was "blown to pieces," killed by a booby trap.

He recalled that his battalion lost nine men in a firefight forty-five days prior to his departure from Vietnam. He remembered listening on the radio to air strikes against American troops. He stated that the only serviceman with whom he kept in contact with after his discharge, Don Stryker, died from "cancer amputation of his right leg." Further, he stated that although he previously had alleged that he had received a Bronze Star, he had been confused and had actually received an Army Commendation Medal. In the final sentence of his statement, the appellant wrote: "If you need more information please let me know."

JUDICIAL APPRAISAL

In April 1991 the RO sent a letter detailing the appellant's claimed stressors to the U.S. Army and Joint Services Environmental Support Group (ESG) in order to attempt to verify the alleged stressors. A report of the ESG, dated May 1991, stated: On March 4, 1968, LZ Crystal received heavy mortar and recoilless rifle fire resulting in light damage; elements of the 2nd Battalion, 22nd Infantry, participated in combat operations in Cambodia during May and June 1970; PFC Russell D. Wake died from a self-inflicted gunshot wound at LZ Uplift on July 7, 1969; and Specialist Fourth Class Donald F. Webb was killed in action on March 9, 1970. The ESG was unable to document an enemy ground attack at LZ Crystal during the period February 1 through April 30, 1968. The ESG also could not confirm how Specialist Fourth Class Webb was killed. The ESG stated that in order to be able to research the other stressors that the veteran mentioned, more specific information was required from him. The record on appeal, however, does not indicate that the RO ever requested that supplemental information from the appellant.

In a rating decision dated July 1991, the RO again denied service connection for PTSD. After recounting the appellant's claimed stressors, the various diagnoses of PTSD, and the findings of the ESG, the RO determined that the veteran's records did not contain evidence of verified stressor events.

The RO noted that appellant's Army Commendation Medal was awarded for meritorious achievement rather than for valor in combat. The RO also noted that although the ESG had verified the suicide of PFC Russell Wake and the death of SP4 Donald Webb, these incidents were not sufficient stressors to warrant a finding of PTSD. With respect to those instances where the appellant indicated that he had witnessed other soldiers near him being killed in combat, the RO concluded that he had not provided sufficient information to allow verification by the ESG. The RO provided a Supplemental Statement of Case in August 1991. In its decision dated April 21, 1992, the BVA denied appellant's claim for entitlement to service connection for PTSD. A timely appeal to the CAVC followed.

Mr. Zarycki's was a major appeal case on the court's calendar that would require a three-judge panel. The outcome of this panel's review is law. In return, the Secretary of the Department of Veterans Affairs will be held accountable to the court that each level affected by the decision will comply with the findings. One question that comes to mind is: if the Secretary instructs his Board of Veterans Appeals and all Regional Offices to comply with the CAVC's rulings, why does the VA continue to fail to acknowledge any legitimate claim?

COURT'S RULING
Here is what the court had to say in the matter of *Alex E. Zarycki v Brown*:

A. Breach of Statutory Duty to Assist
The BVA found that appellant's claim for service connection for PTSD was well grounded and that the VA had satisfied its duty to assist appellant in developing the claim. After carefully reviewing the evidentiary record, the Court agrees that appellant fulfilled his initial burden of submitting a well-grounded claim; as noted in Part I,

the record contains several diagnoses of PTSD by VA neuropsychiatrist, psychiatrists, and psychologists, including one psychiatrist who noted that appellant was "overtly anxious when he was talking about his Vietnam experiences" and another psychologist who noted that "lying just beneath the surface is a great store of combat mayhem themes." In addition, the record contains appellants lay statements and hearing testimony to the effect that he had been engaged in combat with the enemy and had been exposed to significant stressors during his service in Vietnam.

Because appellant's claim for service connection for PTSD was well grounded, the Board was required to assist him in developing the facts pertinent to his claim. Contrary to its findings in its decision, however, the BVA did not carry out its statutory duty to assist.

Although the Environmental Support Group (ESG) was unable to document all of the information supplied by appellant related to his alleged combat experiences in Vietnam and the alleged stressors he experienced during that period of service, it was able to verify some of the information. Further, and more importantly, the ESG informed the VA that it required additional information from appellant in order to investigate further his claimed experiences in service. Despite the fact that appellant had volunteered to provide additional information if needed, the record contains no evidence to suggest that the VA ever requested such information from appellant. In failing to accept appellant's offer and to afford him the opportunity to respond to the ESG's request for additional information, the VA breached its statutory duty to assist appellant in developing his claim.

The breach of the duty to assist takes on additional significance in the context of this appeal because the BVA did not make a specific factual finding as to whether or not appellant was "engaged in combat with the enemy." Instead, the board appears to have intertwined the issue of whether appellant was engaged in combat with the enemy with whether there was corroborative evidence of his alleged in-service stressors:

A valid diagnosis of [PTSD] requires, first of all, that there be a confirmed service stressor. American Psychiatric Association: *Diagnostic and Statistical Manual of Mental Disorders* 250 (3rd ed., revised, 1987.) When referring to combat situations, there must be corroboration that the veteran was exposed to more than the ordinary stressful environment of a combat zone. We are not bound to accept either the veteran's uncorroborated account of his Vietnam experiences or a psychiatrist's unsubstantiated post-service opinions that the veteran's alleged [PTSD] had its origins in service.

The veteran's DD Form 214, Report of Transfer or Discharge, does not list any decorations that would indicate actual combat. Although the veteran initially contended that he won a Bronze Star, he later withdrew this contention. There are no complaints or findings in service of a psychiatric disorder, and the first post-service evidence of a psychiatric problem was not until April 1983, when the veteran was hospitalized because of the stress of a divorce, alcohol use, financial difficulties, and his inability to find a job.

Although PTSD was subsequently diagnosed, this diagnosis was based on the veteran's subjective history. His contentions that his unit was involved in a ground attack on LZ Crystal in March 1968 could not be verified by the [ESG] which did determine that LZ Crystal received heavy mortar and recoilless fire resulting in light damage in March 1968. Additionally, the veteran's contentions that he was in an armored personnel carrier in approximately June 1970 that was ambushed, resulting in several deaths, could not be verified. Since there is no independent evidence confirming that the veteran was exposed to more than the ordinary stress inherent in service in a combat zone, service connection for PTSD is not warranted.

On remand, appellant will have the opportunity to provide the VA with the supplemental information requested by the ESG. Appellant is reminded that "the duty to assist is not always a one-way street. If a veteran wishes help, he cannot passively wait for it in those circumstances where he may or should have information that is essential in obtaining the alleged evidence" (duty to assist fulfilled where two attempts were made by VA to obtain necessary information despite the limited data supplied by appellant).

After fulfilling its duty to assist, the BVA then will have the opportunity to make a specific factual finding as to whether or not appellant was engaged in combat with the enemy based on all the evidence of record. The Board will support its finding with an adequate statement of reasons or bases. If the BVA determines that appellant was engaged in combat with the enemy and that appellants alleged stressors are related to such combat, appellant's lay testimony, without further evidentiary development, will be enough to establish the occurrence of the claimed in-service stressors provided that such lay testimony is satisfactory, credible, and consistent with the circumstances, conditions, or hardships of such service.

The BVA will then need to determine (1) whether appellant's claimed stressors are sufficient to support a diagnosis of PTSD, i.e., *events during service that are outside the range of usual human experience and that would be markedly distressing to almost anyone,* and (2) whether appellants currently diagnosed PTSD is causally related to those stressors.

If the BVA finds that appellant was not engaged in combat with the enemy, or that appellant was engaged in combat with the enemy but that his claimed stressors are not related to such combat, it then will have to determine, as a preliminary matter, whether appellant's testimony as to the claimed stressor is corroborated sufficiently by service records to establish the occurrence of the claimed stressful events (case remanded for BVA to address whether appellant was engaged in combat with the enemy, to examine the circumstances, conditions, and hardships surrounding his period of service, and, if necessary, to corroborate the occurrence of his alleged service-related stressors). Next, the BVA will have to determine whether the claimed stressful event is a sufficient stressor to support a PTSD diagnosis and whether appellant's current PTSD is related to the claimed in-service stressful episode.

B. Additional Arguments

Before this Court appellant contends that the BVA erred by misapplying the diagnostic criteria for 1150 in the DSM-III-R; specifically, he posits that to support a diagnosis of PTSD stemming from a claimant's military service, a stressor must consist of exposure to "more than an ordinary stressful environment" rather than "more than the ordinary stressful environment of a combat zone," as stated by the BVA in its decision. Appellant essentially contends that service in a combat zone may, in and of itself, constitute a sufficient stressor to support a diagnosis of PTSD. For the reasons discussed in before appellant's contentions are without merit.

Appellant also asserts that the BVA erred in (1) basing its decision on the opinions of one psychiatrist rather than a board of two psychiatrists as the BVA had previously directed in its December 1990 decision; (2) rejecting the medical diagnoses supporting appellant's claim based on its own unsubstantiated medical conclusions; (3) failing to give due consideration to appellant's lay testimony; and (4) failing to apply the benefit of the doubt doctrine.

Because the BVA determined that there was no evidence of in-service stressors, however, it never reached the issue of whether or not appellant currently suffers from PTSD, irrespective of whether or not it would be related to service. As a result, the BVA did not address the medical evidence and lay testimony supporting appellant's current diagnoses of PTSD, did not rely on any medical evidence to support its decision, and did not discuss the application of the benefit of the doubt doctrine. However, in view of the need for a remand for readjudication, there is no need for the court to address these arguments at this time.

A remand is meant to entail a critical examination of the justification for the decision. The Court expects that the BVA will reexamine the evidence of record, seek any other evidence the Board feels is necessary, and issue a timely, well-supported decision in this case.

Upon consideration of the record and the filings of the parties, the court finds that a remand is warranted. Accordingly, the Secretary's improvident motion for summary affirmance is DENIED, the BVA's April 21, 1992, decision is VACATED; and this matter is REMANDED for further proceedings consistent with this opinion.

This case demonstrates that an appeal may not be concluded for years and also shows how court members think.

Chapter 9: What Have We Learned?

1. Military personnel who serve in combat zones and do not have a combat MOS (such as infantryman) must meet a higher standard of proof to qualify for PTSD benefits. As this case shows, the veteran was part of a combat-unit but because he was assigned as a wireman and switchboard operator, his word was not acceptable under 38CFR 3.304(f) to trigger further development by the VA. As the case illustrates, the RO did not know what to ask for beyond requesting more hard evidence.

2. The VA in this case relied on SMRs and DD-214 as the basic review records in denying the veteran's claim. They are supposed to obtain detailed information concerning the veteran's combat unit history.

   The director of the Veterans Benefits Administration issued a letter to all VA Regional Offices and centers on January 8, 2001, which dictates they must make every effort to obtain all pertinent evidence, including private medical records, the veteran may have referred to, before they make an unfavorable decision.[10]

3. Regional Offices do not follow the remand order issued by the Board of Veterans' Appeals. They pretty much do what their own operational policy dictates. This makes it critical that you review your copy of the BVA's remand order making certain the local RO is in compliance. If not, immediately file a Notice of Disagreement, stating their determination is flawed.

4. According to the APA's *Diagnostic and Statistical Manual of Mental Disorders, 4th edition*, a valid diagnosis of PTSD requires, first of all, that there be a confirmed service stressor. When referring to combat situations, there must be corroboration that the veteran was exposed to more than the ordinary stressful environment of a combat zone.

   You can preempt the possibility of your PTSD claim being denied if you contact the Environmental Support Group, now known as the U.S. Armed Services Center for Research of Unit Records, and request pertinent information concerning your circumstances under the provisions of the Freedom of Information Act.[11] You can also search the web for after action reports by typing "after action reports" into any search engine.

5. Once you have developed a detailed list of combat incidents that supports your contention of PTSD caused by a combat-related stressor, contact your local congress member or senator to forward your request to USASCRUR.

   When a member of the congress forwards a request, government agencies go into overdrive to respond.

6. One of the first things that should strike you about this case is the number of years it takes to get a PTSD claim through bureaucratic mine fields. To

succeed you must be light-years ahead of the VA by anticipating exactly what evidence you need to establish a well-grounded claim and what evidence you need to fully support your claim.

7. If you have been awarded any one of the medals listed in M21-1MR, part IV, subpart ii, chapter 1, section D, paragraph 13 and have been diagnosed as being disabled by PTSD you have met the combat standard, therefore, you do not have to provide additional evidence to start the claim process.

8. To write a statement of all your experiences, the outline of Sgt. David Raz's sworn statement to the VA is a good example.

9. If you can possibly obtain a psychological evaluation prior to submitting your claim for PTSD you will have a much greater influence on the outcome of your claim.

10. Do not submit any evidence that cannot be verified. This is especially true if the root of your trauma is not combat related. The six court decisions provide an excellence guide on what to do and what not to do.

11. The first basic step is to submit an informal claim. It protects your early entitlement date but gives you a year to put your claim together with all the necessary evidence.

12. It's essential that you go back and reread the "What We Learned" sections after each of the appeals in this chapter. Look at them as the dos and don'ts in preparing your PTSD claim.

Notes

1. *Barela v. West*, 11 280 (Vet. App. 1998).
2. *Flayter v. Principi*, 2 409 (Vet. App. 1992).
3. Key knowledge for any veteran seeking a hearing before the U.S. Court of Appeals for Veterans Claims is that there are two basic types of decision the court renders. When a three-judge panel decides a case, the findings are binding on the veteran and the Department of Veterans Affairs. This means that if you are in a similar situation you can cite that case as precedent and the VA must rule according to the finding of the court. However, if the decision is rendered by a single judge, the decision is only applicable to that case and cannot be used as a binding decision in similar cases.
4. *William F. Allen v. Anthony J. Principi*, 237 F.3d 1368 (3rd Cir. 2001).
5. *William F. Allen v. Anthony J. Principi*, CAVA Docket Number 01-298, April 27, 2004.
6. *Yancy v. Principi*, Docket Number 01-298, April 27, 2004.
7. *Doran v. Brown*, 6 Vet. App. 283 (1994)). (*Robert E. Doran v. Jesse Brown*, USCAVC Docket No. 93-228 March 8, 1994.)

8. *Alex E. Zarycki v. Jesse Brown*, 6 91, 98 (Vet. App. 1993).
9. The summary of this case has been edited to clarify points and to remove references to legal aspects that are not of interest for our purposes.
10. Robert J. Epley, Training Letter Based on PTSD Review, January 8, 2001.
11. The U.S. Armed Services Center for Research of Unit Records can be found online at http://www.tpromo.com/usvi/claims/step2.htm.

GLOSSARY

affidavit	A written statement that is sworn before a notary public. When the claimant, family, or friends provide such testimony, the VA must accept the statement as evidence and give it proper weight.
Agency of Original	The VARO where the claim first adjudicated.
AOJ	agency of original jurisdiction
appeal	A request for a review of an AOJ determination on a claim.
appellant	An individual who appeals an AOJ claim determination.
Armed Forces	U.S. Army, Navy, Marine Corps, Air Force, and Coast Guard.
board	Board of Veterans Appeals.
board member	A law judge appointed by the Secretary of Veterans Affairs and approved by the president, who decides veterans' benefits appeals.
BVA	Board of Veterans' Appeals. The VA department that reviews benefits claims appeals and that issues decisions on those appeals.
Central Office	The Director of the Compensation and Pension Service, VA Central Office, shall approve all VA regional office determinations establishing or denying POW status with the exception of those service departments findings establishing detention or internment was by an enemy government or its agents.
claim	A request for veteran's benefits.

claim file   The file containing all documents concerning a veteran's claim or appeal.

claim number   A number assigned by VA that identifies a person who filed a claim; often called a "C-number."

Court of Veterans Appeals
                                  An independent United States Administrative Court that reviews appeals of BVA decisions.

date of receipt   The date on which a claim, information, or evidence was received in the Department of Veterans Affairs, except as to specific provisions for claims or evidence received in the State Department or in the Social Security Administration of Department of Defense as to initial claims filed at or prior to separation.

decision   The final product of BVA's review of an appeal. Possible actions are to grant or deny then benefit or benefits claimed or to remand them back to the AOJ for additional action.

determination   A decision on a claim made at the AOJ. (Local Regional Office).

discharge   Separation including retirement from the active military, naval, or air service.

evidence   Records, documents, exhibits, or any probative material introduced to support your claim.

fair preponderance   Evidence that must be sufficient to prove that the evidence against the veteran's claim outweighs that evidence offered in support of the claim.

file   To submit in writing.

former prisoner of war
                                  A person who, while serving in the active military, naval, or air service, was forcibly detained or interned in the line of duty by an enemy or foreign government, the agents of either, or a hostile force.

hearing	A meeting, similar to an interview, between an appellant and an official from the VA who will decide an appellant's case, during which testimony and other evidence supporting the case is presented. There are two types of personal hearings: regional offices hearings (also called local office hearings) and BVA hearings.
hostile force	Any entity other than an enemy or foreign government or the agents of either whose actions are taken to further or enhance anti-American military, political, or economic objectives or views or to attempt to embarrass the United States.
in the line of duty	When an injury or disease is said to be "in the line of duty," it means it was incurred or aggravated during a period of active military, naval, or air service unless such injury or disease was the result of the veteran's own willful misconduct or, for claims filed after October 31, 1990, was a result of his or her abuse of alcohol or drugs. A service department finding that injury, disease, or death occurred in line of duty will be binding on the VA unless it is patently inconsistent with the requirements of laws administered by the VA.
issue	A benefit sought on a claim or an appeal. For example, if a claimant submits an appeal of a decision on three different matters, the appeal is said to contain three issues.
marriage	A marriage valid under the law of the place where the parties resided at the time of marriage, or the law of the place where the parties resided when the right to benefits accrued.

non-service-connected

With respect to disability or death, such a disability was not incurred or aggravated, or that the death did not result from a disability incurred or aggravated, in line of duty in the active military, naval, or air service.

notice	A written notice sent to a claimant or payee at his or her latest address of record.

Notice of Disagreement

> A written statement expressing dissatisfaction or disagreement with a local VA office's determination on a benefit claim that must be filed within one year of the date of the Regional Office's decision.

political subdivision   Includes the jurisdiction defined as a state and the counties, cities, or municipalities of each.

preponderance of evidence

> Demonstration that the VA's evidence is superior to that which was introduced by the veteran before a claim may be denied.

probative evidence   Evidence that has a tendency to prove or actually prove an alleged entitlement.

proximate cause   An event that caused an injury or disease and without such injury or exposure the disability would not have occurred.

reasonable doubt   In a VA claim action, the term implies certainty that must be applied before benefits can be denied. If the amount of evidence for and against the claim is equal or nearly equal, the decision must be in favor of the claimant.

Regional Office   A local VA office; there are fifty-eight VA Regional Offices throughout the United States and its territories.

Regional Office hearing

> A personal hearing conducted by an RO hearing officer. A Regional Office hearing may be conducted in addition to a BVA hearing.

relevant   Refers to evidence that is pertinent, relative, connected to the point or target.

remand   An appeal returned to the Regional Office or medical facility where the claim originated.

service connection   With respect to disability or death, that such disability was incurred or aggravated, or that the death resulted from a disability incurred or aggravated, in the line of duty in the active military, naval, or air service.

state Each of the several states, territories, and possessions of the United States, the District of Columbia, and commonwealth of Puerto Rico.

Statement of the Case (SOC)

Prepared by the AOJ, this is a summary of the evidence considered, as well as a listing of the laws and regulations used in deciding a benefit claim. It also provides in formation on the right to appeal an RO's decision to BVA.

Supplemental Statement of Case (SSOC)

A summary, similar to a SOC, that the VA prepares if a VA Form-9 contains a new issue or presents new evidence and the benefit is still denied. A Supplement Statement of the Case will be provided when an appeal is returned (remanded) to the RO by the Board of Veterans' Appeals for new or additional action.

traveling board hearing

A personal hearing conducted at a VA Regional Office by a judge of the BVA.

veteran of any war Any person who served in the active military, naval, or air service during a period of war.

veteran service organization

An organization that represents the interests of veterans. Most veterans' service organizations have specific membership criteria, although membership is not usually required to obtain assistance with benefit claims or appeals.

war time service The following dates are formal periods of war. If a veteran served during one or more of these periods, he or she will have been considered as serving during a wartime period: WWI, April 6, 1917–November 11, 1918 (Veterans who served in Russia between April 6, 1917–July 7, 1921 are also considered wartime veterans);

WWII, September 16, 1940–December 31, 1946;

Korean Conflict, June 27, 1950–January 31, 1955;

Vietnam War, August 5, 1964–May 7, 1975 (If you served as an advisor in Vietnam, any time between February 28, 1961 and August 4, 1964);

Persian Gulf War, August 2, 1990 to a date yet to be determined.

Wartime service also means any time in which combat service was performed during between January 1, 1947 and a date yet to be determined. Several examples would be the Berlin Air Lift, Lebanon Crisis, Grenada, Iranian Crisis, and Bosnia.

waters adjacent to   With regard to service during the Mexican boarder period, the waters (including the islands) that are within 750 nautical miles (863 statute miles of the coast of the mainland of Mexico).

willful misconduct   An act involving conscious wrongdoing or known prohibited action (*malum in se* or *malum prohibitum*). A service department finding that injury, disease, or death was not because of misconduct will be binding on the Department of Veterans Affairs unless it is patently inconsistent with the facts and the requirement of laws administered by the Department of Veterans Affairs.

INDEX

ABOUT THE AUTHOR

John Roche's involvement as a veteran's advocate began nine years before he retired from the U.S. Air Force. His VA actions on behalf of retired military personnel came to the attention of the St. Petersburg Regional Office's adjudication officer when, as a causality assistance officer, he successfully argued for a widow that her retired Air Force officer husband's accidental death in the county jail was service-connected.

Immediately after leaving the air force, Roche joined the VA Regional Office adjudication division as a claims specialist. During the three years that he was with the VA, he completed its 1,560-hour formal training program and gained considerable insight into why so many claims were denied. Veterans did not know how to prove their claims; they relied on the VA to do it for them.

His decision to leave the VA was fostered by policies that contradicted the reason he accepted the job. Since leaving the VA, Roche has used his knowledge of the system to help more than forty thousand clients during the past thirteen years as a county service officer. Health reasons caused him to step down as an active veteran's advocate with the county service in 1996.

Roche is a published writer specializing in veteran's issues and has four forthcoming books on the subject. He has written five books focusing on how to get claims approved. His books have introduced him to veterans from all over the United States who have had legitimate claims denied.

Mr. Roche is a lifetime member of the Disabled American Veterans, National Association of Uniform Services, and the Military Officers Association of America. He is also a member of Congressman Michael Bilirakis's advisory board. He lives in Palm Harbor, Florida.